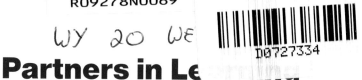

WY 20 WE

Partners in Learning

A guide to support and assessment in nurse education

Ian Welsh

and

Caron Swann

Radcliffe Medical Press

Radcliffe Medical Press Ltd
18 Marcham Road
Abingdon
Oxon OX14 1AA
United Kingdom

www.radcliffe-oxford.com
The Radcliffe Medical Press electronic catalogue and online ordering facility.
Direct sales to anywhere in the world.

British Library Cataloguing in Publication Data

A catalogue record for this book is available from the British Library.

ISBN 1 85775 555 3

Typeset by Aarontype Ltd, Easton, Bristol
Printed and bound TJ International Ltd, Padstow, Cornwall

Contents

Preface

The importance of the need for clinical nurses to be involved in the education of nursing students has been emphasised by the English National Board for Nursing, Midwifery and Health Visiting (ENB) and the Department of Health (DoH).[1] For many years the ENB Course 998 Teaching and Assessing in Clinical Practice has been the main course of preparation for this role; however, as the nature of nurse education has changed a new form of preparation has been considered necessary. This has been influenced by government health policies reflected in such publications as *Making a Difference*,[2] and *The NHS Plan*.[3]

A variety of terms have been used to refer to the role which nurses have undertaken in supporting students, recognising the multiplicity of functions it entails; the ENB/DoH have decided that the term *mentor*, an all-encompassing term, is appropriate. This term is derived from Greek mythology and refers to a wise and trusted guide. The purpose of this book is to help you use your accumulated nursing wisdom in a trusting and mutually respecting relationship with your students. It is intended to be of use for nurses undertaking the Mentorship Preparation Programme, although we hope that more experienced mentors will also find it of value.

The idea for this book came about during a planning and review meeting to discuss a short course, entitled Teaching and Assessing in Clinical Practice, which we were running at Liverpool John Moores University. As news came through that this course was to be phased out we considered that such a text would still be necessary for its replacement course. It was felt that the texts we were using at the time were either too academic, in the sense that they focused mainly on theoretical aspects of nurse education, or that they were too basic and did not offer the clinical nurse sufficient guidance in the rich opportunities that were available for teaching in clinical practice. So we sat down and brainstormed our ideas about the ideal book.

As we noted our thoughts it became apparent that to be of any value to practitioners we should take a pragmatic approach – whatever guidance we give about teaching nursing must be practical – usable in the context of the busy clinical environment; something that will ultimately result in clinical competence for the nursing students who are taught by registered nurses. However, in keeping with the current values in nursing, it is not enough to simply provide a manual – a 'how to do it' book. Any ideas we propose need to be based on strong academic foundations. In an era of evidence-based practice it would be negligent of us not to offer some support for our ideas, however as experienced teachers and practitioners we have developed our own insights and techniques into education which we have found to be effective. Our evidence base therefore, may just be ourselves and we offer no apology for this. It has been argued by Welsh and Lyons[4] that the intuition of experienced practitioners may be as valuable as evidence based on randomised controlled trials. In fact we would go so far as to say that you should develop your own techniques and, if they work, stick with them. This book offers a wide range of ideas on many aspects of nurse education but, at best, books can only be guides, their value lies in what you, the reader, develop from them.

The second principle was that we should keep the language simple; we have no intention of 'talking down' to our readers but we are conscious that every profession generates its own language, or jargon, and education is no different from any other. We aim to explain our ideas so that you know what we are trying to say. Writing a book should not be about showing people how clever we are, it is about communicating – just like teaching really.

Our motivation for writing the book at this time was two-fold. First, we believe that there is a need for a pragmatic book, and second because the British Government is emphasising the need for partnerships between the National Health Service (NHS) and higher education institutions (HEIs), hence the word 'partners' in the title. However, after submitting our outline proposal to the publisher, various reviewers, including some from abroad, suggested that we aim for an international readership. One of the difficulties inherent in a task like this is that we are writing as British nurse educators working in the UK and inevitably we are influenced by the context in which we are working; we also wish to contribute to the partnership in education ideal, as discussed above. Nevertheless, we believe that many of the aspects of clinical education we are addressing are relevant to clinical nurse educators in any social or national context.

While we have been teaching our course it has become apparent that not all practitioners are committed to taking a teaching role. It is not uncommon to hear comments such as 'we are too busy to teach' or 'our job is to nurse patients, not teach your students' or even 'teaching is your job, you should come out here and do it'. Comments like this indicate a number of things – the pressures and stresses of clinical nursing, the tension between education and practice and a lack of practitioners' ownership of professional education. While we certainly agree that patient care is the primary responsibility of the practitioner, the view that they have no responsibility to teach needs to be explored. In the UK it has long been accepted (in principle if not always in deed) that practitioners should teach, and this is reflected in salary and clinical grading criteria. Nevertheless there is a real tension between the expectation to deliver patient care and to teach students. For some practitioners the solution is to opt out of teaching, for others it is to attempt both tasks and suffer from role strain. The publications, in the UK, of *Fitness for Practice*[5] and *Making a Difference*[2] have emphasised the need for partnerships in education, with NHS Trusts and HEIs working together to develop students who will meet the employment demands of the service. As a result of these reports pre-registration nursing education is undergoing an overhaul to iron out some of the problems which resulted from the radical change in pre-registration education when the apprenticeship system was abandoned in 1989, in favour of the Diploma in Higher Education (Dip HE) course, commonly known as Project 2000. One of the problems identified was the increasing division between education and practice as nurse education left its NHS base for the universities. To address this problem the reports recommend the development of strong partnerships between NHS Trusts and HEIs, where each recognises the strengths and potentials of the other in the enterprise of preparing students for entry on to the professional register. As a result the Dip HE curriculum is being rewritten and developed in NHS and HEI partnerships, with partnership agreements clearly stating the sharing of this responsibility. (Our own institution is, in fact, one of the lead sites which has been chosen to develop this initiative.) However, legal documents do not alter individuals' perceptions and there is still much work to be done to persuade many practitioners of their contribution to nursing education. We would argue, in relation to this, that if nurses do not prepare people for their own professional register someone else will. One feature of a profession is that it regulates its own membership. One of the authors is old enough to have taken his written qualifying examinations by answering a paper set, in part, by doctors, following a course in which doctors' lectures featured prominently. If the nursing profession is not bothered about who it is that prepares and assesses its entrants then it does not matter if nurses refuse to accept teaching and assessing roles. It is our belief that nursing has so many features which are uniquely different from its related professions that the people best qualified to teach it, and to assess students' fitness for practice, are the practitioners themselves. We recognise the strain that this imposes, but if clinical teaching and assessing could be viewed as belonging somewhere on the patient care continuum, perhaps the tension might be reduced. For example, if a high standard of patient care is really important then it makes sense to ensure that everyone giving care is properly educated for their role. Nursing students give care; by not teaching them how to do it practitioners are contributing to low standards of care. We are suggesting, therefore, that the notion of caring should extend to caring about what and how students are taught in clinical practice. As practitioners you have expertise in the art and science of nursing, which is what your students want to learn from you. You have the potential to add the skill of effective teaching to your professional repertoire, which will not only improve the quality of care for your patients now but also for your students' patients in years to come.

At this point it may be worthwhile considering who your students are likely to be. It is all too easy to class students under a broad stereotype, say as young and female, with only one aim – to learn nursing and get on to the professional register, or to acquire an additional professional qualification. In fact nursing students are as different as any other group of people. Some are relatively free of other responsibilities, some may be older students with dependent relatives. Degrees of interest, competence and confidence may vary considerably, as may personal backgrounds. A small scale study by Kelcher[6] showed that some students experienced severe hardships, often unrelated to their nursing courses, and succeeded by virtue of hard work, tenacity and sheer determination to be a nurse. Sometimes students tell us that the qualified staff supervising them were not interested in them, that they were seen as just a pair of hands, and not very useful ones at that. We believe that students will respond to the effort that you put into their education and that having made the commitment to learn nursing they are keen to take advantage of every opportunity to learn from the experts. We hope that as you read this book, and work through the exercises, you will gain not only the skills of clinical teaching and constructive assessment, but also the enthusiasm to share the highly rewarding business of improving patient care through education, whether it be in pre- or post-registration courses.

This book is called *Partners in Learning* because we believe that effective nurse education can only come about through a true partnership of the concerned parties – practitioners, academics and the students themselves. Strong partnerships are characterised by respect for each others' needs, a willingness to help each other without being unduly critical of perceived weaknesses, and a clearly defined mutual aim. We hope to show, in this book, how practitioners and academics can work with students to enable them to be capable of delivering the highest quality of care which people with health needs require.

Ian Welsh
Caron Swann
School of Health and Human Sciences
Liverpool John Moores University
November 2001

References

1 ENB/DoH (2001) *Preparation of Mentors and Teachers: a new framework for guidance.* English National Board for Nursing, Midwifery and Health Visiting and the Department of Health, London.

2 DoH (1999) *Making a Difference: strengthening the nursing, midwifery and health visiting contribution to health and healthcare.* DoH, London.

3 DoH (2000) *The NHS Plan.* DoH, London.

4 Welsh I and Lyons CM (2001) Evidence based care and the case for intuition in clinical assessment and decision making in mental health nursing. *Journal of Psychiatric and Mental Health Nursing.* **8**: No. 4.

5 UKCC (1999) *Fitness for Practice.* UKCC, London.

6 Kelcher A (2000) *Getting Through*: the lived experience of student nurses. Theme paper, Nurse Education Tomorrow. Eleventh Annual International Participative Conference, University of Durham, September 2000.

About the authors

Ian Welsh B Ed (Hons), RGN, ONC, Dip N (London), RNT
Principal Lecturer
School of Health & Human Sciences
Liverpool John Moores University

Caron Swann M Ed, Cert Ed, RNLD
Senior Lecturer
School of Health & Human Sciences
Liverpool John Moores University

About the contributors

Bridgit Dimond MA, LLB, DSA, AHSM, Barrister-at-law
Emeritus Professor
University of Glamorgan

Bob Swann MEd, MBA, RMN, CPN Cert, Cert Ed
Clinical Governance Co-ordinator
Guild Community (NHS) Trust
Preston

Acknowledgements

In writing this book we have been indebted to a number of people for their help in various ways. The encouragement and support of Andrew Bax, Managing Director of Radcliffe Medical Press, and Paula Moran, Editorial Co-ordinator, whose patience showed no bounds, has been invaluable. The unknown reviewers of our draft provided us with stimulating thoughts, and showed us the value of peer review. We are also grateful to Imogene Foster, Associate Professor at the West Virginia University School of Nursing, USA, for her comments in the early stages. For her contribution to the legal aspects of assessment, Bridgit Dimond deserves a special acknowledgement for stepping in at short notice. And to Keith Hornby, nursing student at the School of Health and Human Sciences, Liverpool John Moores University, our appreciation for allowing us to use his reflective account in Chapter 7.

Finally, a word of thanks to our families who put up with our long absences while we were closeted away writing, and particularly to Clare Welsh who took some of the typing workload off her dad for a mere pittance of a payment.

A note on terminology

A decision was made very early on in the production of this text to adopt the English National Board's (2001) definition of *mentor*:

> 'The term "mentor" is used to denote the role of the nurse, midwife or health visitor who facilitates learning and supervises and assesses students in the practice setting.'

In addition to this we attempted to avoid using gender specific language whilst at the same time trying to side-step cumbersome combinations such as his/her, etc. Where masculine or feminine pronouns have been used, it is not intended to imply that a person of that gender is the usual occupant of the position referred to.

During the preparation of this book my wife became seriously ill. Her recovery is due to the quality of care she received from a wide range of health professionals at the Royal Liverpool University Hospital, and we will always be grateful to them. The book is intended to promote excellence in nursing care and this could not have been demonstrated better than by that which Helen received on Ward 9A and in the Intensive Therapy Unit. Jan Wyness, Joan Taylor and Karen Ravenscroft deserve a special mention for their professionalism in a crisis. This book is for you all.

Ian Welsh

CHAPTER ONE

The changing face of nurse education

Chapter overview

- Review of the development of nurse education
- The social context of nurse education
- The transition from the product to process approach to education
- Project 2000 and beyond
- Integration of theory and practice
- The relationship between higher education principles and occupational standards
- UKCC outcomes and competencies

There have been many criticisms of the changes to nurse education since it moved from its traditional hospital base into higher education. This chapter aims to put this change into context in the hope of explaining why it had to occur. It should not be regarded as a definitive historical account; it is more a collection of thoughts from the author, who has been involved in this field, since the 1960s, as a student, clinician and educator. The 1960s were a defining time for western society: this was a period when social conventions, class divisions and the authority of established institutions, such as the church, were all called into question. As a result of these factors, many changes in the infrastructure of society also changed, partly due to the need to adapt to the new society, and partly because the people involved in the infrastructure were themselves part of the changes. Nursing was slow to adapt, preferring to evolve gradually, but technological and political changes forced the profession to rethink its provision to the public. Consequently, nursing education, in some parts of the western world, underwent a major reorganisation. This chapter outlines this development referring, when necessary, to related changes in other institutions and ways of thinking, and concluding with reference to educational development at the beginning of the third millenium.

What does the social revolution of the 1960s have to do with nurse education now?

Prior to the social revolution in the 1960s, social convention and conformity were established features of western society. Educational achievement was very much class-related, higher education being the preserve of the more affluent upper middle classes. The idea of people 'knowing their place' in society was subtly instilled by the establishment; for example the Christian children's hymn *All Things Bright and Beautiful* contains the words 'The rich man in his castle, the poor man at his gate, God made them high and lowly, and ordered their estate'. Through such subliminal messages people knew where they stood in society's pecking order. There were those born to govern, those born to manage, i.e. carry out the orders from above, and the majority, whose role it was to carry out the instructions of the managers. As a consequence, trainees in vocational courses such as nursing were, by today's standards, not very well educated and more willing to accept the direction of their superiors.

In the UK, since it was formalised in the 1920s, nursing education followed a pattern which consisted of transmitting existing knowledge and demonstrating clinical skills. The student was expected to accept these unquestioningly and learn them by rote, a method of vocational training which reflected the needs and values of western society up until the 1960s. The social revolution of the 1960s dramatically affected the established order and the younger generation not only questioned, but also challenged conventions. The deference of previous generations was abandoned; consumers demanded rights and patients wanted information in order to understand their medical conditions and to make informed decisions regarding treatments. These changes were reflected in the way educationalists saw their function. The traditional role of schools and colleges was to prepare pupils for their place in a largely pre-ordained workforce, in other words to create a 'product', to be used by employers. The 'product' model of education is one in which there is a clear definition of what the student is expected to learn, learning being demonstrated by the ability to recall facts and reproduce the skills which had been taught in a programme of instruction. This approach does not require the student to understand the underlying principles behind the knowledge or skills; like experimental animals they simply have to reproduce the required responses. As a method of training this is actually quite effective; the teacher has control over what is to be taught, the student can learn by rote, without having to struggle over complex concepts, and assessment is simply a matter of answers being right or wrong.

How did the social revolution affect patients' attitudes?

The social hierarchy pervaded all strands of society, including the health sector; if a person became ill they were expected to submit their minds and bodies to the superior knowledge and skills of the medical profession. Compliance was expected by health professionals and given by the patients. The American sociologist Tallcot Parsons summarised this in his classical observation on the 'sick role' when he noted that ill people are tolerated by their family, employers and significant others only if they seek and accept medical advice.[1]

Nurses trained under the traditional system would be able to perform quite effectively with a compliant patient group; however, as more people were becoming aware of their rights as consumers they demanded information on which they could base their decisions regarding medical treatment. No longer were they likely to accept a doctor's decision to medicate or operate unless they knew of the alternatives or the possible unwanted effects of treatment. The professional group with whom patients spent the most time was, as now, nurses, and it was inevitable that patients would seek information from them. Nurses were seen by many as a primary source of information, someone to consult if they had no information, or as a secondary source if they wished to obtain further information after being spoken to by a doctor. The traditional training of nurses had failed to prepare them for this sort of role and it was recognised by the profession that a different approach to the preparation of nurses was needed, one which not only gave them the facts and manual skills which were necessary for patient care, but also the intellectual skills to understand the theoretical basis of their profession, the ethical issues involved and the knowledge to discuss health issues with their patients.

How did the nursing profession respond?

The history of nurse education is characterised by resistance to significant change. Davies described changes in this field as 'a series of small concessions slowly gained but no real challenge ... to the basis of nurse education'.[2] Clay referred to the 'triumph' of gradualism, meaning that while education developed it did so only if the students could continue to contribute to ward staffing.[3] The role of hospital matrons was discussed by Spouse, in relation to their control of nurse training as a means of ensuring an adequate source of labour on the wards.[4] The opportunity in 1972 to respond to societal changes, and significantly change education, was offered in the publication, by the British Government, of the Report of the Committee on Nursing (the Briggs Report).[5] However, the opportunity was lost because of '... the profession's public disarray during the passage of the Briggs Bill.[3] Clay noted that the profession was so engrossed in tearing itself apart that it failed to notice that Parliamentary time was running out. Consequently there was not sufficient political will among nursing leaders to create the changes which would enable the profession to respond appropriately to the demands created by the social revolution.

However, among nurse educators, there was a realisation that the product approach had severe limitations, and subtle changes were brought into teaching methods. These were largely influenced by the work of Stenhouse,[6] who described a 'process' approach to education. This differed from the product-centred curriculum in that it emphasised the development of the individual by concentrating on students' ability to understand underlying principles. Take for example the question: *'Should a patient with chronic lung disease be given high or low concentration oxygen?'* There is only one correct answer, which is low concentration, but being able to recall it does not provide any evidence that the student understands *why* this is the correct answer. Nurses are no longer people who simply carry out doctors' instructions; they have to develop nursing care plans which reflect the needs of individual patients. Intelligent nursing requires an understanding of the disease process in relation to normal anatomy and physiology, or 'normal' human behaviour. In this example, therefore, the nurse who does not understand why a high concentration of oxygen would be dangerous to the patient will not have a clear understanding of physiology or the disease process. If the nurse cannot understand what the disease is doing to the patient then he or she is likely to see only a person with a set of symptoms. Responding appropriately, sometimes in an emergency, requires the ability to identify problems and apply solutions, not merely to act in a reflex way.

The realisation that nurse education needed to change eventually led to the publication, in the UK, of a series of consultation papers from the United Kingdom Central Council for Nurses, Midwives and Health Visitors (UKCC), culminating in the overwhelming support from the nursing profession for the introduction of a curriculum based on the principles outlined in *Project 2000, A New Preparation for Practice.*[7]

This change mirrored developments in other parts of the western world; in New Zealand the publication of the 'Carpenter Report' resulted in the transfer of nurse education from hospital-based schools of nursing to diploma-level courses based in polytechnics.[8] In the early 1980s in Australia, nurses literally took to the streets to demonstrate their support for change. Consequently, in 1985 their hospital-based courses gave way to diploma-level courses in higher education institutions (HEIs).

Despite the the fact that the profession had demanded changes, reactionary voices objected, expressing concern that nurses at the point of registration were not as competent as those trained in the apprenticeship system. The response of the UKCC to these views was to establish a commission, under the chairmanship of Sir Leonard Peach; its remit was 'to prepare a way forward for pre-registration nursing and midwifery education that enables fitness for practice based on healthcare needs'. The outcome was the publication of the report *Fitness for Practice.*[9] One of the conclusions reached was that the reforms of 1986 showed that students 'have well developed skills in critical reasoning', and 'are better able to adapt to change and implement evidence-based practice than those trained under the old, apprenticeship style model'. Despite the fact that there was still doubt about their level of practical competence, no substantive evidence for this belief was offered in the report. The publication *Making a Difference* expressed the view that nurse education should be more competence-oriented, and this document was instrumental in bringing about another major curriculum review.[10] A small number of nursing schools within the universities were chosen, by the Department of Health, to be lead sites, that is to say they had to develop competence-focused curricula which were to be implemented by the autumn of 2000. The majority of the rest of the schools were to implement their changes by 2001, and the remainder by 2002.

Has the wheel turned full circle?

Cynics would argue that Project 2000 had failed, and that the attempt to raise the intellectual level of nursing had been achieved only at the cost of losing the clinical skills, which were at least guaranteed under the apprenticeship system. However, the question has to be asked, if students were really not as competent as they ought to have been, how did they manage to qualify when qualification partly depended on their ability to demonstrate proficiency in clinical skills in each of the clinical areas in which they worked? Clinical assessment was undertaken by clinical nurses, not by academics. (*See* Chapters 4 and 5 for further discussion on this issue.)

Interestingly, neither *Fitness for Practice*,[9] *Making a Difference*,[10] nor *The NHS Plan*[11] have suggested that nurse education should revert to its lower academic level, so the principle of the 'knowledgeable doer' still stands. Perhaps rather than saying that the wheel has turned full circle, it would be more accurate to say that curriculum development is an upward spiral process, in which issues are revisited and developed in the light of objective evaluation. It is important to note that educational systems are not entities that exist in isolation from the rest of the world, they are both a product and a tool of the societies that they serve. As society has developed from being compliant and deferential to being more assertive and demanding of information, nursing education has had to ensure that the nurses it produces are capable of meeting the challenge. The product approach to education could only produce nurses who responded in a limited, reflexive way. The process approach produces nurses who have a deeper understanding of the scientific, social and psychological principles on which their practice is based.

How does course design achieve the new objectives?

In the UK, diploma and degree courses are structured to enable the student to build on previous learning, a significantly different approach to the previous system. Prior to the introduction of Project 2000 a conventional study programme would consist of a number of short study blocks which focused on medical conditions. A typical study block outline is shown in Table 1.1.

Table 1.1 The outline of a study block

Topic	Content
e.g. Urology	Anatomy and physiology of the genito-urinary system Medical conditions of the genito-urinary system Surgical conditions of the genito-urinary system Relevant nursing care Pharmacology relating to the genito-urinary system

There was no difference in the academic level of learning from years one to three, the only difference being in the content of the study blocks. Also there was no significant assessment of the psychological or sociological aspects of illness, which meant that there was no significant input. The revised approach within the diploma courses enabled the students to build on their basic knowledge. Figure 1.1 illustrates academic progression, which clearly shows the differences expected at various stages of the course.[12]

At the beginning of the course the student learns the basic knowledge at a deeper level than students on the previous apprenticeship courses. Deeper means having the ability to explain why and how, rather than merely the ability to recall what. For example, in physiology the answer to the question '*What is the hormone which controls carbohydrate metabolism?*' would require a simple recall answer – insulin – without testing the student's understanding of the answer. A test of comprehension might be something like: '*How does insulin control the metabolism of carbohydrate?*' When the student has mastered the knowledge and comprehension elements of the course they progress to the level of analysis. This higher level cognitive ability is one in which students can review a set of information

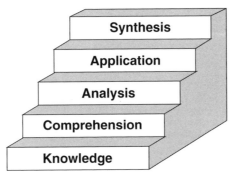

Figure 1.1 Academic progression.

and use their understanding of the relevant principles to make a judgement on it. This might be information in a book or journal, or it might be the symptoms and clinical history with which a patient presents. Take, for example, a situation in which an elderly person has been admitted to the ward showing evidence of neglected personal hygiene. Knowing that poor hygiene can result in ill health of some sort, the student might be inclined to tend to the patient's immediate needs, such as bathing and care of the hair and teeth. The analytic student would first ascertain the reason for neglect, to see if it was due to a physical inability to undertake self-care as a result of illness, or if it was due to depression and a lack of will on his part. Having ascertained this, the decision can then be taken to apply the knowledge and skills which are relevant to this particular patient. The process of synthesis is one of constructing a plan of care to meet the patient's needs based on the analysis of available information.

This broad outline of progression is based on the modular system, a more sophisticated system of course design than that which was used in traditional nurse training schemes. Many HEIs use this approach to curriculum design, although there are those who take the slightly different approach of segmenting learning into units. Whichever method is used, the principle is that students undertake discrete sets of learning activities, which must build on each other. Learning from earlier modules, or units, is an essential prerequisite for further learning, and the student is able to make relationships between modular or unit contents.

Is the modular approach counterproductive to effective learning?

One problem of the modular system is that it may encourage some students to take an instrumental view of their course. Progress is perceived to be a matter of 'passing modules'; once a module has been successfully completed the student mentally sets it aside to focus on the next one. Rust describes the process as '. . . a series of hurdles to be jumped and forgotten'.[13] This demonstrates the conflict between the intentions of the educationalists and the students. No matter how noble the aims of the educationalists, the students will more often than not be focused on doing whatever is necessary to pass. Consequently this provides a challenge to curriculum planners to develop a course which will achieve its educational aims, not just in setting up a 'series of hurdles to be jumped', but to make sure that the route is interesting enough for the students to want to explore the areas between the jumps. In other words, to encourage the students to focus on learning, rather than on assessment. This might be achieved by addressing another concern, that of the gap between theory and practice, remembering that the context of this curriculum review is a perceived dissatisfaction, by health service employers and nurses, with the outcomes of the educational reforms resulting from the UKCC document *A New Preparation for Practice*.[7]

Conventionally, curriculum development tends to focus on content and strategy, i.e. what should be taught and how it should be delivered. It would be missing the point if, in addressing this dissatisfaction, we were not to give prominence to assessing the competencies which, it is claimed, are lacking. The main concern seems to be that, at the point of registration, nurses are not competent to practice. If this is the driving force for change then it follows that the assessment of students must feature strongly in curriculum planning. Assessment may seem to be an afterthought, once the content and strategy have been determined. In an academic programme of preparation for registration, students will undertake a wide variety of learning in academic and practical settings. The breadth and depth of learning encompasses a range of subjects and fields of nursing. This multidimensional aspect of learning needs to be assessed in a variety of imaginative and, for the student, constructive ways without an over-reliance on extended essays and clinical assessments of dubious quality. The really important aspects of professional and academic development cannot be assessed unless there is some agreement on what those competencies are which need to be assessed.

The purpose of Project 2000 was to develop 'knowledgeable doers', an aphorism denoting nurses who were to be competent practitioners with the academic skills needed to understand and develop their practice. Unfortunately, after ten years, the perception is that while the intellectual dimension of nursing has been addressed, the practical dimension has suffered. By including assessment as an integral part of curriculum planning, and not relegating it to the latter end of a teaching and learning process, the result should be nurses who are fit for practice, fit for purpose and fit for academic awards.

The *Fitness for Practice* report recommends a 'competence–outcomes-based curriculum'.[9] This is consistent with the direction in which higher education is moving, according to the Quality Assurance Agency for higher education* (QAA). QAA recommend that course design should be based on an outcomes-based learning (OBL) model.[14] Jackson describes the benefits of this, in relation to professional education such as nursing. In discussing the sharing of academic and occupational standards he says that 'the design intention of an integrated system is that it facilitates access to, and progression through, the learning opportunities provided in ways that more compartmentalised systems cannot'.[15]

Rust acknowledged the danger that modular programmes encourage compartmentalisation by students who do not always look for connections between modules, or who cannot see the relevance of one to another.[13] The OBL model could perpetuate this unless the requirements of the professional bodies are clearly incorporated within the course. QAA assessment guidelines make it clear that 'institutions should ensure that ... clear information is available to staff and students about specific assessment requirements that must be met for progression toward the professional qualification'.[16]

Incorporating professional standards into an academic framework

If modular programmes have the potential to lack cohesiveness, then some way must be found to ensure that modules do link together, and are dependent on each other. In 2001 the UKCC provided a list of outcomes and competencies which must be achieved in order for the student to gain professional registration (*see* Appendix). Four 'domains' were identified as being essential for registration purposes:[17]

- professional and ethical practice
- care delivery
- care management
- personal and professional development.

---

* The QAA is an organisation established in 1997 'to support higher education institutions in discharging their responsibility for the quality and standards of their educational provision'.

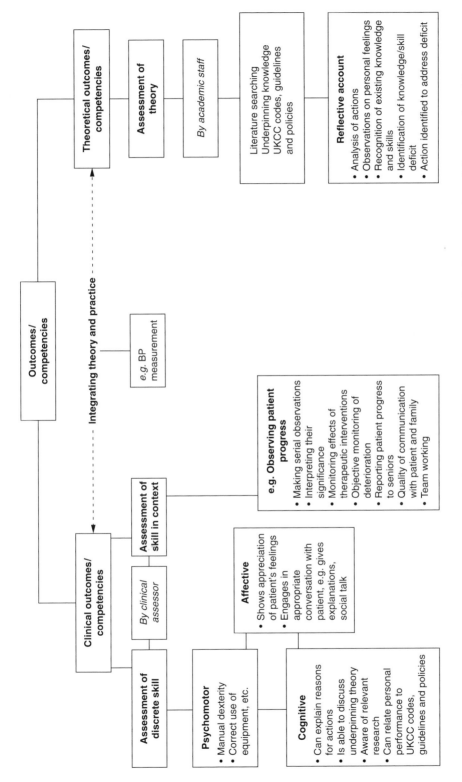

Figure 1.2 A portfolio of evidence of achievement of outcomes and competencies to show the integration of theory and practice.

These requirements are consistent with the OBL principles, in that there are clear statements of 'what is to be learned'. The domains are broken down into two levels – outcomes and competencies. Progression occurs when the student achieves the outcomes required for successful completion of the foundation programme, and moves into the branch programme (i.e. adult, child, learning disability, mental health). It continues when the student achieves the competencies in each domain, putting them in a position where they can apply for professional registration. The terms outcomes and competencies simply refer to end points, or targets to be achieved. In QAA terms this will be demonstrated through the assessment of 'what is actually learned'. Because the targets are rooted in clinical practice but have theoretical bases they are not easily separated from each other, thus providing the cohesion necessary to make a successful modular programme.

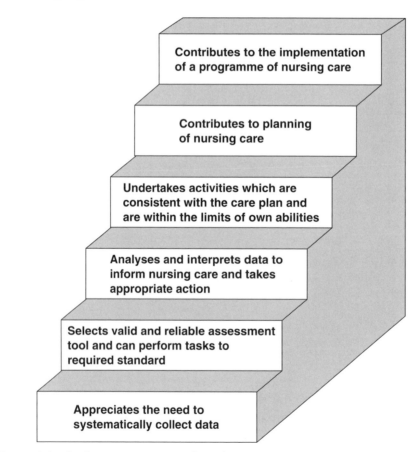

Figure 1.3 Student progression in clinical practice.

It might be helpful to see how this breaks down, using one particular nursing skill as an example. Figure 1.2 illustrates how, by taking the example of blood pressure measurement, students are encouraged to explore what is to be learned from a variety of perspectives. Assessment would be by a collection of evidence (a portfolio) showing clinical and academic achievement.

As the student acquires a range of assessment skills he or she can begin to contribute to the identification of patient needs and the development and implementation of an effective care plan, within the parameters of the UKCC outcomes and competencies. Figure 1.3 shows student progression based on the outcomes for care delivery at foundation programme level. This model will be used in Chapter 3 to help you to develop your own teaching strategies.

This sequential development assists student motivation by helping them to value their own contribution to nursing care, and to develop the skill of identifying their own learning needs, as a basis for negotiated learning supported by clinical supervisors and academic staff. If we add to this the component of professional and ethical practice, it can be seen that each of the UKCC domains have been used, at least in part. This then provides the cohesion required for a successful modular programme.

Summary

The preparation of nurses has evolved from a task-focused training into an educational system which aims to develop students' intellectual ability as much as their clinical competence. The need for this arose from changes in the expectations of society, and the form of care which was required by a more critical and questioning client group. The transition has not been entirely without its problems; comparisons between the perceived level of competence between traditionally-trained nurses and those who undertook diploma-level courses have led to doubts being expressed about the clinical competence of diplomates and graduates at the point of registration. To some the gap between theory and practice, which already existed in the traditional system, has widened as nurse education moved into the higher education system and away from its hospital base. The response, in the UK, has been to create a competence-based framework, within a programme of academic study, to ensure that the original aim of developing knowledgeable doers could be achieved. By developing stronger partnerships between clinicians and academics, NHS trusts and universities, and between professional bodies and universities, it is hoped that the theory–practice gap will be effectively bridged.

References

1 Parsons T (1951) *The Social System.* Routledge and Kegan Paul, London.

2 Davies C (ed) (1980) A constant casualty. In: *Rewriting Nursing History. Nurse Education in Britain and the USA to 1939.* Croom Helm, London.

3 Clay T (1987) *Nurses: power and politics.* Heinemann, London.

4 Spouse J (1900) *An Ethos for Learning.* Scutari Press, London.

5 HMSO (1972) *Report of the Committee on Nursing.* HMSO, London.

6 Stenhouse L (1975) *Introduction to Curriculum Research and Development.* Heinemann, London.

7 UKCC (1986) *Project 2000, A New Preparation for Practice.* UKCC, London.

8 WHO (1971) *An Improved System of Nurse Education for New Zealand.* New Zealand Department of Health, Wellington.

9 UKCC (1999) *Fitness for Practice.* UKCC, London.

10 DoH (1999) *Making a Difference.* DoH, London.

11 DoH (2000) *The NHS Plan.* DoH, London.

12 Bloom BS (1956) *Taxonomy of Educational Objectives: the classification of educational goals/ Handbook 1: cognitive domain.* Longman, London.

13 Rust C (2000) An opinion piece: a possible student centred assessment solution to some of the current problems of modular degree programmes. *Active Learning in Higher Education,* Vol. 1, No 2. Sage Publications, London Institute of Learning and Teaching.

14 QAA (1999) *A Consultative Paper on Higher Education Qualifications Frameworks for England, Wales and Northern Ireland (EWNI) and for Scotland.* Quality Assurance Agency for Higher Education, Gloucester.

15 Jackson N (2000) Programme specification and its role in promoting an outcomes model of learning. *Active Learning in Higher Education,* Vol. 1, No 2. Sage Publications, London Institute of Learning and Teaching.

16 QAA (2000) *Code of Practice for the Assurance of Academic Quality and Standards in Higher Education, Section 6: assessment of students.* Quality Assurance Agency for Higher Education, Gloucester.

17 UKCC (2001) *Requirements for Pre-registration Nursing Programmes.* UKCC, London.

CHAPTER TWO

Teaching with confidence

Chapter overview

- The act of learning
- Examining your own teaching experience
- The need for structure in teaching
- Planning a lesson
- Lesson delivery
- The interpersonal aspect of teaching
- Applying psychological learning theories

Introduction

In the previous chapter we referred to the need to develop stronger partnerships between clinicians and academics to reduce the gap between theory and practice. One way of doing this is to share the responsibility for the education of students. As a nurse with expertise in your own particular field of nursing you have a great deal to offer the next generation of nurses which can complement the theoretical learning taught within the classrooms of the universities.

One of the frequently stated aims of course participants on our Teaching and Assessing in Clinical Practice courses has been to improve their confidence in teaching. When we ask if they can nurse confidently they are invariably quite positive; this would suggest that although they are happy with the *content* of their lessons, they appear to be diffident about their *method* of teaching. Essentially, good teaching is a combination of the teacher having a sound grasp of the topic and the ability to deliver it effectively. The aim of this chapter is to help you to organise what you know, and can do, into a format that will help you to communicate it to your students.

Although planning and organisation are essential requirements for teaching, we believe that two overriding principles should be at the heart of every teacher: the first was best expressed in the words of Carl Rogers, an influential humanistic thinker, who stated that 'teaching is a vastly over-rated activity'.[1] If this seems a little strange to include in a chapter on teaching it is important to add that he went on to say that this is only the case if the teacher believed that his or her aim was the transmission of knowledge. He also said that 'teaching isn't important, learning is'. The focus of a teacher's activity must be the student's learning; teaching may seem, by some, to be an ego trip – an opportunity to show off all that we know, or can do. How much good this does for the student is debatable, certainly some learning can take place, but this puts learning as a passive process, with the student simply receiving information, whereas deeper learning is an active process, one in which the student is actively involved, and not merely a spectator. In this chapter we intend to use this principle by encouraging your active participation through exercises designed to develop your teaching ability. We want you to learn *how* to teach rather than to learn *about* teaching, so try to avoid skipping the exercises and be prepared to spend time and effort on them: it should help you to become a more effective teacher.

Activity 2.1

Can you recall being taught by someone who is more concerned about showing off their own knowledge/skill than about helping you to learn?
What were your feelings towards the session?
What evidence of learning could you demonstrate afterwards?

What happens when we learn?

When learning is taking place there is an increase in the production of chemical transmitter substances in the brain, which makes the synapses more efficient at transmitting signals. When the learning circuit has been completed it only requires a trigger to set off the circuit to enable us to recall the information, or skill, that we have learned.[2] This is why when we have taken the trouble to learn something, for example how to play a musical instrument or the rules of a game, we only need slight prompting to recall the skill. Compare this with an occasion when you were being taught, but not actually paying attention, and try to remember how 'permanent' that learning was. Our memory is the store of information which we have learned, which enables us to recall information or to repeat skills without having to relearn them each time. A useful model (or representation) of memory is the Atkinson-Schiffrin model (Figure 2.1).[3] This shows how some information is stored successfully and some is not.

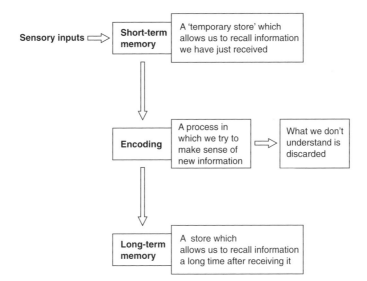

Figure 2.1   The Atkinson-Shiffrin model of memory.

This model of memory attempts to explain how we remember things, and also how we can forget them. We are bombarded every second with sensory inputs; so stop for a moment and try to focus on the information that you are receiving *now* via your five senses. This tells you what is happening *outside* your body, so also focus on what your body is telling you about *inside* your body. Have you any discomfort, aches and pains, is your bladder full? Without looking are your knees straight or flexed?

All of this sensory information is coming at you while you are trying to learn from a lecture, textbook or demonstration, and *all of it* goes into your *short-term memory*. That is to say, every second you are gaining a mass of information, most of which you do not need, for example the sensations you experience during a clinical demonstration, such as traffic noise or the smell of fresh paint, have no relevance. All sensory inputs are then *encoded*. We try to give them meaning; those which have no relevance now are discarded. Can you remember the traffic noise during your demonstration? If you can understand a new piece of learning, i.e. it makes sense to you, and you can give it meaning in relation to your own experience, then you have successfully *encoded* it and it will enter and remain in your *long-term memory*. If you can't make sense of it, it will not be retained. Only information stored in the *long-term memory* can be recalled. Memory, therefore, is very much dependent on learning, making sense of information, and making sense is an active process. This is why 'teaching is a vastly over-rated activity'. It is learning that is important. By participating in the learning process yourself you will develop a greater appreciation of the need to help your students to learn, as opposed to being taught.

You as the teacher

This section is intended to help you look at yourself as the teacher, in order to identify your positive attributes in this field. It will also help you to recognise where you may wish to develop, so that your teaching can become more effective. Because teaching is an individual activity the best way to review yourself as a teacher is to reflect on some of your recent teaching sessions. The activities below are designed to guide your thoughts; reflection is an activity which, when done well, can lead to vastly improved performance through the development of new insights.

Activity 2.2

In what ways have you been involved in teaching students in the last few weeks?

1 Working with them
2 Demonstrating a skill
3 Explaining a concept
4 Discussing patient care
5 Other (describe briefly)

How do you know if your teaching was successful or not?

What personal qualities do you have which contributed to your teaching?

On reflection, what aspects of your personal development do you feel you need in order to improve your teaching?

Activity 2.3

What feelings do you recall having *during* your last teaching session?

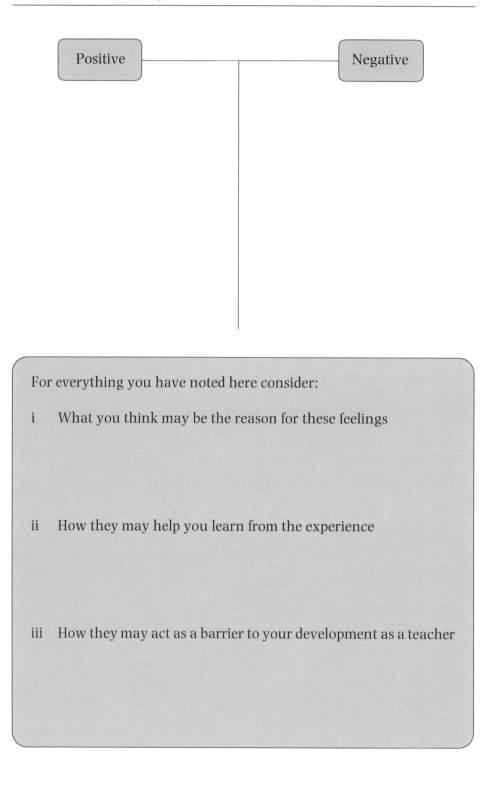

| Positive | | | | Negative |

For everything you have noted here consider:

i   What you think may be the reason for these feelings

ii   How they may help you learn from the experience

iii How they may act as a barrier to your development as a teacher

It may be helpful, at this point, to read the notes written by a former student, who reflected on a lesson she gave. In her reflective diary she wrote:

> *'Felt confident . . . however, it was a disaster . . . it became clear I had knowledge gaps.'*
> *'Another session . . . same topic as my "disaster", but this time I had updated and researched . . . I maintained control . . . the problem was that I hadn't allocated enough time.'*

These brief notes indicate some common failings among new teachers, an overconfidence in their grasp of the theoretical content, and flaws in the planning of the lesson. Sometimes it is only when we try to teach something that we realise that we are not as clever as we like to think!

Activity 2.4

Review the strengths and weaknesses of your recent teaching.

Grade yourself on a scale of 1 to 5 (5 being high) on the following:

I was confident with the *content* of my teaching (i.e. the knowledge or skill being taught)   1 2 3 4 5
Make a note of your strengths and weaknesses here:

I was confident with my *teaching method.*   1 2 3 4 5
Make a note of your strengths and weaknesses here:

Planning your teaching

This section is about structuring your teaching, that is to say it is concerned with developing your teaching method. Teaching is often a spontaneous activity, especially in busy clinical settings, which is where students learn almost all of their clinical skills. You could, therefore, reasonably ask if developing a structure for your teaching is a practical proposition. We want to make it quite clear that we are not suggesting that you divorce your teaching from the normal activities of your workplace, nor are we attempting to replicate a university classroom situation amid the hustle and bustle of your ward or department. What we are proposing is that you develop a framework within which to operate, perhaps in the same way that you use a framework in certain clinical situations.

Activity 2.5

What do these situations have in common?

1 When a patient collapses you automatically begin a sequence of events, such as checking the airway, breathing and circulation. You call a doctor, get resuscitation equipment, etc.

2 When working with a group of clients you notice that one is showing signs of agitation. You fear that a violent incident might occur and immediately take steps to defuse it by tactfully removing the client from the group and attending to his problem, while at the same time ensuring your own personal safety.

Although both are very different circumstances, they each require the experienced nurse to recall and implement an effective stategy, in other words a framework for action. Teaching may be planned or spontaneous; you may decide in advance that you are going to demonstrate a skill at a particular time of your shift, or you may decide as you are doing something that this would be an appropriate opportunity to demonstrate the skill to your student. In either case, a teaching framwork can make your teaching more efficient.

> ## Box 2.1
>
> Consider these notes from the reflective account of another of our students. She wrote: '*Upon reflection . . . the sessions were spontaneous and relevant . . . however, the lack of structure and preparation must have led to omission of details.*' In these statements she is showing insight into her own development needs, particularly the need to learn how to plan her teaching. After working on this aspect she improved her 'mental framework', that is to say, she gave herself a structure in which to work. Her progress was subsequently shown in a diary entry where she described a teaching session given at a time of staff shortages when she and her student were both tired. She wrote: '. . . *some positive aspects were identified – learning outcomes gave a more structured feel and having notes to hand reduced the risk of omissions.*' However, she also noted: '*Overall there was minimal student activity . . .*' The notes of her next session stated: '*Encouraging greater interaction with students seemed to facilitate a more humanistic approach, as the sessions were more student-centred.*'

These notes suggest a progressive rate of improvement, and satisfaction, as a result of her reflections and the development of a particular teaching framework. We can now go on to look at some of the principles that contribute to a useful teaching framework.

Specifying a topic

It may seem like stating the obvious, but it is important to determine, at the outset, what you are going to teach. A common mistake made by new teachers is that of being too vague in their intentions. For example, take 'giving an injection' as a topic – do we mean intramuscular, intradermal, subcutaneous or even intravenous? The statement is not clear. The first stage in planning, therefore, is to state concisely and unambiguously what your intention is; this is known as your teaching *aim*. To be clearer, in this example, we could say that the aim is 'to enable the student to give an intramuscular injection safely'. This tells your student quite clearly what you are trying to do; it also focuses your attention on this particular aim and should prevent you from digressing to another subject.

However, stating your teaching aim is rather like saying that you want to reach a certain destination on a journey; although it gives you direction it does not tell you how to get there. Remember also that we said earlier that it is learning that is more important than teaching. Once the aim has been decided it is then necessary to make some clear and unambiguous statements about what it is you want the students to learn, these are known as *learning outcomes* (or sometimes learning objectives). Having stated an aim it is relatively easy to develop the learning outcomes.

A learning outcome is a concise statement of what we expect the student to achieve when the teaching session is over. A lesson plan usually has one aim and a number of learning outcomes (using the travel analogy these are the stages of the journey – when all stages have been completed the destination is reached). Learning outcomes, in order to be most helpful to the student, should have certain characteristics. We will consider the injection example to illustrate the point.

Activity 2.6

Take a look at the following example to see if you can pick out the essential characteristics.

By the end of the day the student will be able to:

1   Select the appropriate equipment.
2   Select the correct drug.
3   Assemble the syringe and needle, using an aseptic technique.
4   Draw up the correct dosage.
5   Ensure that the correct patient is to receive the drug.
6   Administer the injection safely.

Are these outcomes within the students' expected capability, i.e. are they *realistic*?

How can you know if the student has achieved them, i.e. are they *observable*?

Could you say of each task that the students can or cannot do them, i.e. are they *testable*?

Could we reasonably expect the student to learn them, i.e. are they *achievable*?

Can we know if the student can perform the task safely, i.e. is there a clear *standard*?

If you like mnemonics this gives the acronym ROTAS:

Realistic
Observable
Testable
Achievable
Standard

Look back on the learning outcomes in Activity 2.6 to see if they meet the essential characteristics.

Box 2.2

Note that the set of learning outcomes is prefaced by the term 'By the end of the day the student will be able to:'. There are two points to note on this.

1   It denotes a *time* by which the student knows when they are expected to have learned the lesson. This will vary according to the amount or complexity of the learning, or even the opportunity to practise.
2   The term is the *stem* of a number of sentences. Read the stem and any one of the examples in Activity 2.6. It should read as a whole sentence.

With regard to the *observability* characteristic of learning outcomes you will note that each one uses an active verb, for example select or assemble. This is because the only way we can know if someone has achieved the outcome is by seeing if they can perform it. If a student selects a 20 ml syringe to give 1 ml of a drug she or he has made an inappropriate selection (therefore failing this particular 'test'). Mistakes commonly made by new teachers include the use of passive verbs, such as know or understand, as in 'the student will know which syringe to use'. If I say that I know something how can you know what is in my mind? It is only by observing my actions that you could be really sure.

Activity 2.7

Using the essential characteristics shown above select a *skill* that you might teach, and write an aim and learning outcomes.
Look at them critically. Do they meet all of the criteria? Can they be improved while retaining their simplicity?

Activity 2.8

Using the same criteria select a *concept* that you might teach, and write an aim and learning outcomes.
(This might be something like dealing with aggression, or the effects of a drug.)

Did you find it more difficult to write learning outcomes for this last exercise? Some people find it easier to write active verbs for practical skills but harder to do so for concepts. For example, how can we know if a student *knows* the therapeutic and unwanted effects of a drug?

Activity 2.9

An example of a badly written learning outcome is 'the student will be able to understand the therapeutic and unwanted effects of antibiotics'.
Can you turn this into an observable outcome?
Another badly written learning outcome is 'the student will know the problems of prolonged bed rest'. Can you turn this into an observ-

Activity 2.10

By now you should be able to state clear aims and write helpful learning outcomes.
Now select a topic (either a skill or a concept) which you would like to teach and, using the ROTAS criteria, write your aim and learning outcomes.

A note of caution! How many learning outcomes do you have? Why do you think it is not advisable to have more than five or six per lesson?

- Each learning outcome represents an expectation that the student must learn a different item (of knowledge or skill). Too many may create unreasonable expectations, i.e. although individually achievable, in total they may be more than the student can handle at that point in time.
- Each learning outcome represents an amount of time for you to spend teaching. You will need to consider how much time you have; a large number of learning outcomes may commit you to a large amount of time.
- Although we advise about five or six outcomes this is only a rule of thumb, and you may wish to use your own judgement to decide what is best. Some may only represent a small amount of learning, especially if they are not complex concepts or activities. Selecting appropriate injection equipment will not be too taxing, whereas learning how antibiotics work requires the student to master the notions of cell structure, the bactericidal properties of the drug and the concept of the development of resistance.

With practice you will develop the skill of estimating how many learning outcomes are realistic in terms of the student's capacity to learn and your ability to teach in a restricted period of time. If you think that there are too many you could consider breaking the session down into two (or more) sessions.

When writing learning outcomes two other factors need to be considered: what you may expect the student to know already (*prerequisite knowledge*) and problems the student may have in learning the new skills or concepts (*anticipated difficulties*). We can consider these in turn.

Prerequisite knowledge

In Activity 2.6 one learning outcome referred to aseptic technique which presupposes that the student understands the concept of asepsis. You should not be expected to teach the students everything and it is reasonable to expect that they will already have some background knowledge. However, it may be helpful to ascertain that the students do have this knowledge, otherwise they will not be able to achieve the learning outcomes. Conversely, if you assume incorrectly that they do not know something, and proceed to teach it, you risk losing their interest. Ausubel *et al.* made the sensible suggestion that we should ascertain what the student knows, and build on it.[4] This helps the students to extend their existing knowledge, or use it as a basis to develop their skills. In essence we do not teach anything in isolation – the student will always try to relate it to their prior understanding.

Anticipated difficulties

You will know, from your own experiences, that learning is not always easy; sometimes concepts or skills are difficult to grasp. A thoughtful teacher will try to identify those aspects of a lesson which are likely to be difficult, and seek ways to overcome the difficulty. These might include:

- allowing the student frequent opportunities to practice a skill
- using aids to illustrate points, e.g. a diagram to show the location of the sciatic nerve in relation to an injection site.

When we are confronted with a difficult situation we try to make sense of it with all our available resources, particularly our five senses and our intellect (the encoding principle). All the material the student is trying to learn can only be apprehended by the use of the senses, which communicate the 'external' material to the brain. If you think that students may have difficulty with an aspect of your lesson you could think of ways to use some, if not all, of their senses to help them to overcome the problem. The greater the variety of sensory inputs which are used, the more likely the student is to succeed in learning. For example, when teaching cardiopulmonary resuscitation you might tell the student that the sternum should be depressed by about five centimetres. To demonstrate this you could use a manikin, or the students could practise this technique for themselves.

Activity 2.11

- In this example which senses are used?
- How effective would learning be if any one sense was not used?
- If the student could not hear the 5 cm instruction, he or she will not know how far to depress the sternum.
- If he or she could not see the correct positioning of the hands and arms he or she would not be able to perform the skill correctly.
- If he or she did not practise the skill they would not be able to feel the resistance of the rib cage and therefore would not know how much pressure to apply.

Activity 2.12

Referring back to your chosen topic in Activity 2.10:

- What prior knowledge did you reasonably expect your student to have?
- What difficulties of learning might be anticipated?
- How will you try to overcome them?

By this stage in your preparation you will have identified the *resources* you need to teach effectively. You will now need to consider the *time* and the *place* for your teaching.

Time

When thinking about time we need to consider duration and appropriateness.

- *Duration* This will depend on your topic, its nature and complexity. Demonstrating a procedure on a patient sets its own limitations as it would obviously be unacceptable to prolong a patient's discomfort, and should not be repeated on the same patient.

- *Appropriateness* Will you really have time to complete the teaching. Is the student ready to learn this topic at this particular time?

Place

It may seem that the clinical area is the obvious place to teach clinical skills, but is it? As a teacher with responsibility for patient safety you may wish to consider what harm might be done to a patient or client if you were to allow a student to practise on them without sufficient preparation. The skill of encouraging a patient to discuss extremely sensitive issues may be best practised in a role-play situation before allowing the student to do it under supervision with a real patient. Urinary catheterisation requires manual skills which may be better developed using an anatomical model. You may be able to think of more appropriate examples for your own practice.

Activity 2.13

Summarise the ideal conditions for the demonstration of a manual skill.

The teaching area you use should really be one which will allow the student to concentrate on the topic without the distraction of patients calling for attention or colleagues asking for assistance. Informing your colleagues that you will be using an area for teaching should give you the privacy you need. If possible ensure that the student has enough space to observe demonstrations, this is particularly important if a number of students are being taught at the same time. It is also worth remembering that manual skills which are new to the student are learned more easily if the student observes these from the practitioner's side; learning a skill is hard enough without having to learn it back to front. Ask someone to teach you how to knit, or perform some other craft skill, and then sit opposite them to see what I mean.

Delivering the lesson

Whatever topic you are teaching, whether it be a skill or a concept, it will be helpful to decide, in advance, how you are going to deliver your material. All of the issues discussed above represent the background work; it would be a shame to waste the effort by a poor delivery.

Table 2.1 is a worked example of a lesson plan which shows the issues discussed above and how the lesson will be delivered. Delivery is based on the principles of experiential learning described by Steinaker and Bell.[5] In their experiential learning taxonomy they propose five aspects.

- *Exposure*   The teacher demonstrates a skill or explains a concept.
- *Participation*   The student is actively involved in the lesson.
- *Identification*   The student appreciates the need for, or importance of, the material.
- *Internalisation*   The skill or knowledge becomes part of the student's repertoire.
- *Dissemination*   The student can demonstrate by performance or even by teaching the subject themselves.

Activity 2.14

Referring back to your selected topics in Activities 2.7 and 2.8, use the worked example in Table 2.1 as a guide to develop your own lesson plans to teach both a skill and a concept.

Teaching styles

By now you will have prepared two complete lesson plans. These provide the structure for your teaching and will serve as your prompt notes when you are actually teaching. However, they cannot help you in the interaction between your students and yourself. At the beginning of this chapter we referred to the process of teaching as being one which facilitates learning; remember Rogers' statement that 'teaching is a vastly over-rated activity'.[1] As well as having a good set of notes it is important to develop

Table 2.1   Worked example of a lesson plan (for illustrative purposes only)

Topic: Prevention of wound infection

Student information: 2 Dip HE pre-registration students, first surgical placement

Pre-requisite knowledge: Existence of micro-organisms in environment and on self

Justification: Students working on surgical wards need to appreciate the dangers, to the patient, of wound contamination – *identification*

Anticipated difficulties: Students may not understand how micro-organisms interfere with wound healing

Aim: To enable the student to apply the principles of cross-infection in ensuring a safe environment for the surgical patient

Learning outcomes: By the end of the session the student will be able to:
1 Describe the concepts endotoxin and exotoxin
2 Explain how bacterial toxins damage healthy tissue and interfere with the growth of new tissue
3 List the methods of cross-infection
4 Describe the precautions which can be taken to minimise the risk of wound infection

Content	Exposure		Participation	Dissemination
	Duration	Method	Student activity	Assessment
Information on bacterial toxins	5 min	• Refer to students' own experience of infection – spots etc. • Explain why these arose – role of toxins in altering tissues (By helping students to relate the theme to their own experience we are helping them to understand and retain the information – internalisation)	• Describe signs of inflammation which they have observed • Relate signs to action of toxins	Before moving on to next section, ask students random questions on causes of inflammatory signs
'Content' is what we want the student to know or do		'Method' is: 1 how we want to convey the content 2 how we can help the student internalise it	By considering 'student activity' the teacher gives thought to the notion of learning as an active process. Teaching is not just about what the teacher should be doing	The only way anyone can know if learning has taken place is by some outward manifestation, e.g. asking questions, observing practice, observing the student teaching

a rapport between you and your students, which is conducive to learning. Nursing students are adults who will respond positively if treated as such. It can be demotivating if they are talked down to, and they may even feel resentful. One of the teacher's roles is to motivate the student to learn. Although it can be assumed that students want to learn, if the teacher–student relationship is not a good one student motivation may suffer. It is worth considering, at this point, how power relationships might affect the quality of learning. As a qualified nurse you have authority over the students, and as an assessor you are in a position to judge their competence, to the point of influencing whether or not they can continue on the course. The students will be aware of this and will invariably see themselves lower down the hierarchy in relation to you. Some teachers adopt a didactic style, that is to say they see themselves as instructors and, perhaps unintentionally, reinforce the power relationship. It could be argued that there is nothing wrong with a didactic style, as this is simply a reflection of the hierarchy. However, Berne explored the nature of relationships in his discussion of transactional analysis, the process of analysing how people interact.[6] He proposed that individuals have three ego-states: parent, adult and child. These are characterised in Table 2.2.

Table 2.2 Key to transactional analysis terms

Ego state	Examples of characteristics
P = Parent	Caring, critical, nurturing
A = Adult	Rational, prepared to discuss
C = Child	Playful, petulant, compliant

At various times we can adopt one of these characteristics, depending on our current ego-state. For example, if I do not like the way a student is behaving in class I could adopt a 'critical parent' state. If I recognise that a student is trying hard to understand a difficult concept I could adopt a 'nurturing parent' state. Berne maintains that during interactions between two or more people the ego-state of one person will affect that of the others. Figure 2.2 illustrates the effect of a teacher in the critical parent state, while Figure 2.3 shows the effect of the teacher in the nurturing parent mode. In each of these examples the teacher, as the more powerful player, causes the student to respond in a particular way.

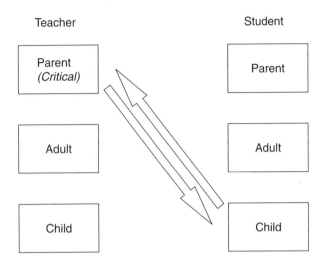

A person in authority who adopts a critical stance is likely
to evoke a response associated with 'child' behaviour,
e.g. resentful, rebellious or subservient.

Figure 2.2   Transactional analysis: the critical parent state.

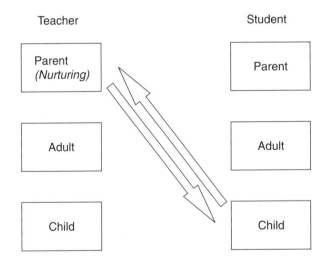

A person in authority who adopts a caring or nurturing stance
is likely to evoke a response associated with 'child' behaviour,
e.g. grateful, dependent, inferior.

Figure 2.3   Transactional analysis: the nurturing parent state.

Activity 2.15

Consider how you might respond in each of the following cases. You have been late for work frequently and your manager says:
1 Your time-keeping is unsatisfactory, come into the office now.
2 Is there anything we can do to resolve your time-keeping problem?

The first situation may cause you to be defensive, while the second situation may encourage you to be open about your problem. In other words, the stance one person takes will evoke a response in another, that is to say, it leads them into another ego-state. While this book was being written a General Election was about to take place in the UK. At one stage during the electioneering process someone threw an egg at John Prescott, the Deputy Prime Minister; Prescott's response was to retaliate by delivering a punch to the protestor. It could be argued that the egg throwing was the result of a child ego-state, as was Prescott's response. Perhaps it would

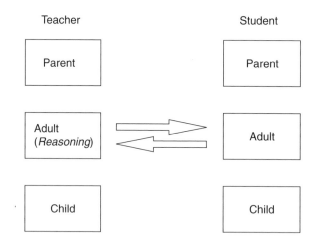

A person in authority who adopts a reasoning stance is likely to evoke a response associated with 'adult' behaviour, e.g. mutually respectful, prepared to consider alternatives, willing to argue reasonably.

Figure 2.4   Transactional analysis: the reasoning adult state.

have been to his credit if the Deputy Prime Minister could have tried to raise the level of the confrontation to an adult–adult one by inviting his aggressor to discuss the issue that prompted his behaviour (Figure 2.4). In the teaching situation the quality of the teacher–student relationship can be enhanced if you take care to treat the student with respect.

Motivation can be enhanced if you take into account the student's own aims.

Maslow described the nature of human motivation as a hierarchy of human needs (Figure 2.5; discussed in Quinn[7]). Maslow proposed that each person had an ultimate goal they wished to achieve and that the goal was their driving force, or motivating factor. In order to self-actualise, or become the person they want to be, a number of needs must be met; failure to meet these needs frustrates the achievement and may be demotivating. Although this refers to personal fulfilment, the principles can be applied to lesser situations. If the pinnacle of achievement in a learning situation is taken to be the achievement of the learning outcomes, the student's other needs must be met. With adult students, we need not be too concerned about ensuring that their physiological needs are met but the teacher can attend to their safety, affection and esteem needs.

Safety needs may include both psychological and physical aspects. Psychological harm, in the sense of damaged confidence, or even guilt, can ensue if the student is allowed to undertake tasks for which they are not adequately prepared, particularly if their actions result in discomfort or harm to a patient. We should not underestimate the anxiety students may have in learning situations, so any care that can be taken to alleviate anxiety will help them to progress towards their goals. In the context of

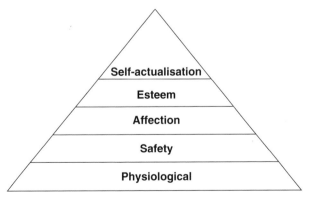

Figure 2.5 Maslow's hierarchy of human needs.

physical safety, students' concerns about prevention of infection or back injuries, for example, need to be addressed by the teacher. When the students realise that the teacher has their welfare in mind they can direct their energies to satisfying their other needs.

The next need, in Maslow's hierarchy, is the need for affection. Affection takes many forms, perhaps in the teacher–student relationship it could be better described as acceptance. Most people have a need to be liked, but what if you do not like your student? Sometimes we just cannot get on with others, maybe because they have personal traits that we dislike, or perhaps because their attitudes or values are different from our own. It should be understood that the teacher–student relationship ought not to be based on likes or dislikes; the nurse–patient relationship is based on the patient's needs, not on personal predispositions. Relationships with students are professional relationships and therefore should be independent of personal feelings. Rogers described the concept of 'unconditional positive regard', that is to say, an acceptance of a person without condition – they do not have to meet your requirements. The notion of acceptance in relation to motivation is discussed more fully in Chapter 6.

Having considered how you can help the students to achieve their goals of safety and affection we can look at the penultimate driving force in Maslow's hierarchy, the need for esteem. Generally we want more than to be just accepted, we seek respect, we want to be valued. Students are at their most vulnerable point when they are moving from their 'comfort zone', where they are at ease with their knowledge, skills and beliefs, to an area of new learning. This is the time when they are formulating new ideas, practising new skills, or are subjecting their existing attitudes, values and beliefs to scrutiny. It is an uncomfortable period of uncertainty where they realise that they are open to criticism. In other words their self-esteem, at this time, might be low. If learning outcomes are not achievable students may believe that they are not capable of succeeding, and become demotivated. The teacher can help by ensuring that learning outcomes are realistic and achievable, and by acknowledging or praising the student's efforts. When this happens the students are aware of the recognition, and even respect, that you are giving them and they have achieved a sense of value. This notion is also discussed more fully in Chapter 6. Although Maslow belonged to the school of humanistic psychology, the idea of positive feedback as a motivator for further learning has its origins in the behavioural psychology school. Skinner believed that students' responses to new situations could be reinforced by such positive rewards as praise and encouragement.[8]

Using psychological theories to enable learning

In the preceding part of this chapter you can see that we have moved from the mechanism of teaching, i.e. preparing lesson plans, to the interactive element, i.e. the relationship between teacher and student. In order to teach effectively it is important to remember the student as a person, not just as an apprentice but as a unique individual with different wants, needs and interests. As unique beings they will also have different ways of learning; some prefer to be instructed; some like to be able to make sense of subject matter by exploring it and developing their own insights; some prefer to learn from their own experiences. In truth, no one is specifically one or the other of these regarding their way of learning; we all have the ability to learn from a variety of ways, but with a stronger predisposition for one method as opposed to the others.

How learning takes place is a topic which psychologists have explored for over 100 years. A number of theories of learning have emerged and it will be useful to look at some of them to see how you might apply them to enable your own students to learn the art and science of nursing.

Behaviourism

As its name implies, behaviourism is concerned with the observable actions (behaviours) of people in the learning process. You can only know if your student has learned if they can demonstrate new knowledge or skills. This school of thought began, not with the work of a psychologist, but with the Russian physiologist Pavlov, whose study on the gastric secretions of dogs is discussed by Atkinson *et al.*[9] This led to the development of his 'classical conditioning' theory after finding that he was able to make his dogs salivate at the sound of the bell, if the sound was associated with food (hence the alternative name associationist theory).

This discovery prompted others to develop the idea that subjects could learn by conditioning, that is to say subjects (i.e. people or animals) could learn to respond in a particular way if certain conditions exist. The Pavlovian method produces reflex learning but a more purposive learning process was described by Thorndike (discussed in Atkinson *et al.*[9]) who demonstrated that appropriate responses could be developed through 'trial and error learning'. One of his experiments involved putting a cat into a box in which a loop of string provided the only means of opening the door. After a series of random actions the cat caught the string and opened the door. Subsequently, when the cat was put into the box, it was able to escape quite easily as it had learned to open the door.

Atkinson *et al.* describe how Skinner developed this idea still further by creating experiments in which animals could learn to perform quite complex actions through a series of behaviours, each of which were rewarded.[9] This is known as 'shaping behaviour', where correct actions are rewarded and incorrect ones are punished. For example, food may be given as positive reinforcement and small electric shocks as negative reinforcement.

Activity 2.16

Can you recall an occasion when you tried to teach someone a skill?

- What did you do when they made a mistake?
- What did you do when they acted correctly?

In professional education we do not use titbits and electric shocks but we do use a range of positive and negative signals. Nods and smiles, sounds of approval and praise are interpreted by the student as indicators that they are performing well. If they unwittingly make mistakes a shake of the head, a sigh or a 'don't do that' are the negative reinforcers that let them know that they are going wrong. The term 'shaping behaviour' is quite descriptive because it suggests that the teacher is sculpting a performance in which the end product is an acceptable level of skill by the student. Features of this approach are:

- teaching is controlled by the teacher
- standards of performance are clear
- all stages of the performance are testable.

Gestalt theory

Gestalt theorists, such as Köhler, Koffka and Wertheimer explain learning as the development of insights. They object to the behaviourist approach because it does not credit the person with the ability to process information and solve problems. Atkinson *et al.* describe Köhler's classical experiments which involved setting problems for chimpanzees.[9] In one instance the animal was in a cage in which a bunch of bananas was suspended beyond reach from the ground. Scattered around the cage were a number of boxes. Köhler observed the chimp at first leaping up, unsuccessfully. It then sat down, apparently doing nothing until it suddenly stacked the boxes on top of each other, climbed up and reached the bananas. Köhler's interpretation was that the chimp was processing the information around it, and then arriving at a solution.

This explanation of learning credits the person with the ability to come to their own conclusions, unlike the behaviourist approach, which is teacher-dominated. An example of this approach in use would be allowing a student to develop a plan of care based on their perceived needs of a patient. Clearly this requires supervision, to ensure that the student does not omit an important aspect, or suggest something which could be harmful, but the teacher is not controlling the student's behaviour. Insightful learning occurs when the student analyses the available information in relation to the patient's problems and attempts to create an appropriate set of therapeutic responses aimed at meeting the patient's needs.

Vygotsky,[10] a cognitive psychologist, developed the notion of a 'zone of proximal development', which refers to the achievement of a child's potential (the *potential* development level) as opposed to their *actual* developmental level. He argued that as 'novices' they could be helped when 'experts' constructed challenging situations that are not so challenging as to be beyond their ability. His notion of 'scaffolding', or constructing a framework, which allows the child to progressively learn something new, is not dissimilar to the care planning situation described above. The term zone of proximal development is important as it refers to the gradual progression of a person's abilities. If the set tasks are too far away from their present state the student can become disheartened and demotivated.

Figure 2.6 illustrates the use of Vygotsky's scaffold theory. The teacher's aims are to help the student to construct a care plan, contribute to care delivery and evaluate the effectiveness of the plan. According to the UKCC's *Requirements for Pre-Registration Nursing Programmes* (UKCC 2001) these are outcomes which should be achieved within the common foundation programme, i.e. within the first 12 months of the course (*see* Appendix). This may seem to be a daunting task to the student but the thoughtful teacher can construct it in such a way as to make it achievable in stages.

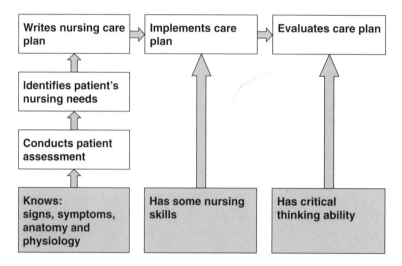

Figure 2.6   A care plan constructed using Vygotsky's scaffold theory.

The shaded boxes represent the student's *actual developmental stages*, the knowledge and skills that they bring to the learning situation. The arrows point to the next item of learning, the *proximal development zone*. As the student develops knowledge and skill in this area this becomes their *actual development stage*, and they move on to the next proximal development zone.

Activity 2.17

By referring to the outcomes in each of the four domains in the UKCC's Requirements for Pre-Registration Programme (*see* Appendix), identify the particular outcomes a student might achieve if they successfully complete this learning task.

Humanistic learning theory

Humanistic theorists take a person-centred view of learning. They argue that behaviourists and cognitivists are both using manipulation to bring about learning. The learning tasks are determined by the teacher and the situations, whether they are behaviour shaping or framework building, are under the teacher's control. Humanists believe that it is the student who should determine what is to be learned, and that learning should relate to their own experiences.

In the introduction to this chapter we quoted Rogers who stated that 'teaching is a vastly over-rated activity'.[1] Humanists see teachers as facilitators of learning, not as the fountain of all knowledge to their students. Rogers believed that people are born with an actualising tendency, that is to say they have a drive that directs them to seek out experiences which will help them to become the person they want to be, which includes developing the professional skills they need to satisfy the work aspect of their being. If a person wishes to be a nurse they put themselves into a position which will enable them to achieve that aim, i.e. they enrol on a nursing course. What they require from you as a professional expert is guidance in gaining the necessary knowledge and skills.

The notion of student-centered learning is the central theme of Kolb's experiential learning cycle.[11] Kolb's view is that a person can learn a great deal if they reflect on their experiences. Figure 2.7 illustrates this process.

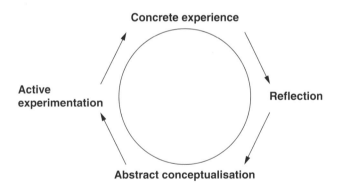

Figure 2.7 Kolb's experiential learning cycle.

This concept will be discussed more fully in Chapter 7.

Social learning theory

If people want to be accepted into a group they have to learn its norms and values, and adopt them as their own. Usually when we join a group we choose one which has norms and values which are congruent with our own. However, when students join a new clinical team on a new placement this choice is not available to them. If they want to gain acceptance into the team (and Maslow indicated that this is an important stage in achieving goals) they will try to ascertain the norms and values of the team by observing, perhaps not consciously, the established group members to pick up cues as to the acceptable ways of acting and, by implication, the attitudes and beliefs of the members.

Melia recognised the importance of this phenomenon in her discussion on the occupational socialisation of nurses. She stated that 'fitting in constitutes a major part of students' behaviour. First they concentrate their efforts on getting on with the ward staff, and second on the actual business of patient care.'[12] Gott cites Asch's study on social conformity and group pressure to show the influence which may be exerted on students to 'toe the line'.[13] Miller observed that 'newcomers in any social situation go through an initial process of learning the ropes: finding out who the other people in that situation are, where they are located, what they do, and how they want him to do it. We seldom dignify this process by calling it learning.'[14] Yet learning it is; insofar as students are picking up the norms and values of the working group to which they have been allocated, there is a learning process going on. It is called adaptation; people who do not adapt themselves to a new environment do not usually thrive in it.

Activity 2.18

Peters' notion of an educated person is described on p. 48. Is social learning compatible with this concept?

What responsibilities does the nurse, as a role model, have?

In order to test the educational value of social learning we can refer to the notion of the 'hidden curriculum'. A curriculum is a set of structured learning experiences with clearly defined content, aims and learning outcomes. Because poor nurses and unsatisfactory clinical teams do exist it is inevitable that from time to time students will be exposed to professionally unacceptable attitudes and practices. Immature students may not recognise these to be poor and may adopt them as their own. However, it is highly unlikely that anyone would say that this is what a student ought to learn, and therefore they would not be stated as curriculum aims.

Nevertheless learning occurs, hence the term hidden curriculum. Because the content (unacceptable attitudes and practices) is not explicit the student learns them unwittingly and cannot be said to be educated in this respect, according to Peters' criteria.[15] There is a responsibility on all practitioners to act in a professionally acceptable manner, firstly for the sake of the patients and clients, and secondly to ensure that the unwitting learning which will occur results in the formation of professionally acceptable attitudes.

Activity 2.19

If social learning occurs as an unconscious process, how can you encourage your students to subject their observations to critical thought?

We suggest that you read Chapter 3 before attempting this activity.

Is there a best learning theory?

As you have read these learning theories it is likely that you have seen something of value in all of them. Perhaps from your own life experiences you have recognised how you have used each one in different learning situations. You may also see, as a teacher, how you could use each of them. In fact you do not have to subscribe to only one school of thought, you can take an eclectic view, that is to say you can use each one as you see fit. Knowles illustrated this in a learning progression graph (Figure 2.8).[16]

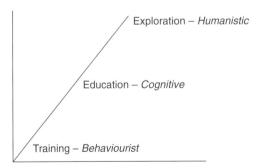

Figure 2.8 Knowles' learning theory continuum.

Learning a task is perceived as a low-level type of learning because it does not necessarily include understanding of underlying principles. In the UK there is a grade of health worker known as the healthcare assistant (HCA). These staff may be trained under the National Vocational Qualification (NVQ) system up to Level 3. At this level they have to demonstrate the ability to perform tasks to a prescribed standard; they do not need to have theoretical knowledge. This is why we have used the word trained as opposed to educated. According to the educational philosopher RS Peters, an educated person is one who has acquired knowledge in depth and breadth, and has done so wittingly.[15] It is possible to pick up skills, snippets of knowledge and even values, beliefs and attitudes without subjecting them to critical thought. Religious or political beliefs may be acquired through indoctrination, for example by being exposed in the formative years to frequent and repeated exposure to the beliefs of close adults or religious ministers. Such a person may be knowledgeable in a narrow field but would not fit Peters' criteria for being an educated person, as their knowledge lacks breadth and has not been acquired voluntarily, but passively. Likewise HCAs, although they may have voluntarily learned a set of tasks, will lack the breadth of knowledge that an educated person would possess.

As we have said, education involves subjecting our learning to critical thinking. A person who is merely trained will perform tasks according to the way behaviour has been shaped. The skill of an educated person can be seen in the way that they adapt their task performance according to their understanding of the situation. A story told to us by one of our students on the teaching and assessing course illustrates this point. An HCA took the blood pressure of a patient as part of a routine observation. The procedure was performed correctly and the result was duly recorded on the patient's chart. Fortunately, very soon after, a qualified nurse saw the patient as she was passing his bed and realised that he was unwell. When she looked at his blood pressure chart it showed a measurement of 80/40 mmHg. The patient was in shock; the HCA had failed to interpret the significance of her observation because she lacked in-depth knowledge. Professional education is more than the mere acquisition of practical skills. It involves gaining a deep understanding of the knowledge which underpins practice (Peters' 'depth' principle). The ability to make connections between seemingly unrelated features is also a requirement for professional practice (Peters' 'breadth' principle). To illustrate this point we could consider the case described by Welsh and Lyons in which a mental health nurse, while conducting an assessment of a patient who had made a suicide attempt, decided not to follow the established protocol and admit the patient to hospital but instead sent him home, having organised community support.[17] This decision was based on her perception that for this patient admission would have created more intolerable problems.

These examples illustrate the cognitive aspect of nursing which cannot be taught using behaviourist techniques. The reason that nursing courses moved into higher education is that Government and the profession appreciated the need to educate rather than to train students. Behaviourist principles have their place in the development of technical skills, but do nothing to develop the insights that are needed for intelligent nursing. Conversely, cognitive principles do relatively little to develop technical skills but are invaluable in developing an understanding of nursing theory. The humanistic approach capitalises on the students' own experiences, and provides a framework for meaningful learning, but it also has its limitations. If teachers did not provide direction regarding material to be learned the novice might not be able to identify their own learning needs.

In summary, behaviourism and cognitivism, being teacher-led, may provide a structure for the student to learn skills and theory, but humanism may be used to enable them to make sense of their experiences in relation to their own existing knowledge, values, attitudes and beliefs.

References

1   Rogers C (1983) *Freedom to Learn in the 80s*. Merrill, London.

2   Myers DG (1995) *Psychology*. Worth, New York.

3   Atkinson RC and Schiffrin RM (1968) Human memory: a proposed system and its processes. In: KW Spence and JT Spence (eds) *The Psychology of Learning and Motivation: advances in research and theory*, Vol. 2. Academic Press, New York.

4   Ausubel D, Novak J and Hanesian H (1978) *Educational Psychology; a cognitive view*. Holt, Rinehart and Winston, New York.

5   Steinaker N and Bell M (1979) *The Experiential Taxonomy: a new approach to teaching and learning*. Academic Press, New York.

6   Berne E (1961) *Transactional Analysis in Psychotherapy*. Grove, New York.

7   Quinn FM (1995) *The Principles and Practice of Nurse Education*. Chapman and Hall, London.

8 Skinner BF (1938) *The Behaviour of Organisms*. Appleton Century Crofts, New York.

9 Atkinson RL, Atkinson RC, Smith EE *et al.* (1996) *Hilgard's Introduction to Psychology* (12e). Harcourt Brace, Florida.

10 Vygotsky LS (1978) *Mind in Society*. Harvard University Press, Cambridge MA.

11 Kolb DA (1984) *Experiential Learning: experience as the source of learning and development*. Prentice Hall, London.

12 Melia K (1987) *Learning and Working: the occupational socialisation of nurses*. Tavistock Publications, London.

13 Gott M (1984) *Learning Nursing: a study of the effectiveness of teaching provided during student nurse introductory courses*. Royal College of Nursing, London.

14 Miller SJ (1970) *Prescription for Leadership: training for the medical elite*. Aldine, Chicago.

15 Peters RS and Hirst PH (1970) *The Logic of Education*. Routledge, London.

16 Knowles M (1984) *The Adult Learner: a neglected species* (3e). Gower, New York.

17 Welsh I and Lyons CM (2001) Evidence based care and the case for intuition in clinical assessment and decision making in mental health nursing. *Journal of Psychiatric and Mental Health Nursing*. **8**: No. 4.

CHAPTER THREE

Critical thinking

Chapter overview

- Introduction
- What is critical thinking?
- How do practitioners develop critical thinking?
- Facilitating critical thinking in others
- Conclusion

Introduction

The introduction to this book makes reference to changes in the preparation of nurses and midwives over the past 80 years. It discusses the move from a product to a process approach in nurse education, outlining progression from an apprenticeship system (traditional training) to the development of the Diploma of Higher Education in Nursing (Dip HE Nursing), commonly known as Project 2000. The previous apprenticeship base delivered training largely of a lower taxonomic level in that student nurses were taught the essential knowledge base, its application and on some occasions gained an understanding as to why they undertook particular tasks. To a great extent, these apprentice nurses rote-learned specific tasks which had associated specific outcomes. Working within a rigid hierarchy, their role was to deliver rather than to question. The profession came to realise one of the shortcomings of such an approach was the perpetuation of existing practice. Practice was rarely questioned and subsequently little, if any, progression was made. In essence, unless an alternative approach was developed, nurses would only ever be able to implement previously learned solutions to problems. What was required was an approach emphasising the process of education; a process which concentrated on providing a rich educational experience rather than a narrower focused programme of training. This latter approach has become a central feature of nursing curricula and strongly influenced the development of the Dip HE (Nursing).

From a clinical perspective the Dip HE (Nursing) promised much for students; supernumerary status offered the opportunity of better supervision; there was less pressure to work and study at the same time plus there was opportunity to consider and question existing practice. However, with hindsight many educationalists and practitioners became unsure as to how far this promise was consistent with reality. This, in turn, led to the publication of *Fitness for Practice*[1] and more recently new requirements for pre-registration nursing programmes.[2] These requirements place incumbent responsibility on educationalists and practitioners to ensure students are prepared to practise both safely and effectively. The programmes are practice-centred and directed towards the achievement of professional competence within a complex and rapidly changing healthcare environment. The overall competencies reflect the need to analyse, critique and use research and other forms of evidence, adapting practice where appropriate. This new preparation of students embraces critical evaluative thinking, which by its very nature takes a process approach. It is not essential to know all of the answers relating to a particular issue or problem. It is much more important to understand the process by which a solution or solutions can be found. Critical evaluative thinking goes a stage further than this, building the capacity or competence to analyse and subsequently synthesise, producing new knowledge and new practices through which care can be improved.

The term competence according to Saxton and Ashworth is overused and ill-defined.[3] However, we must try to provide some degree of definition which aids the development of more common assumption as to its place in current educational provision. The UKCC describes competence as '... the skills and ability to practise safely and effectively without the need for direct supervision ...'[1] It has been suggested that 'Competence is more than knowledge and skill. Values, critical thinking, clinical judgement, formulation of attitudes and integration of theory from the humanities and sciences into the nursing role are also important.'[4] This view is reflected in the UKCC's statement: 'Programmes must ensure that the level of learning must be such as to facilitate the achievement of knowledge, understanding and skill acquisition and also the development of critical thinking, problem solving and reflective capacities essential to complex professional practice.'[1]

This change in thinking has clear implications for clinical staff involved in the preparation of students. The demands of an increasingly complex healthcare system make the ability to think clearly and critically more necessary than ever before. Many practitioners supporting students in clinical practice will have trained under the 1982 syllabus or the 1974 syllabus; each embracing training paradigms which did not emphasise critical thinking, self-reliance, reflective practice or problem solving. Having said this, it is evident that a large number of practitioners, although not specifically trained in these areas, have amassed considerable skill and expertise. However, for some the development of these skills is not necessarily 'second nature' and may need to be developed.

One of the key roles of the mentor is to facilitate the student's reflection and to assist him or her to develop a questioning attitude, the premise of this chapter being that in order to facilitate critical thinking in others, it is necessary to be a critical thinker yourself.

What is critical thinking?

At the outset, it must be acknowledged that it is beyond the remit and capacity of this chapter to examine all aspects of critical thinking or to examine any one aspect in great depth. It is our intention, therefore, to provide an overview of some of the key aspects of critical thinking. According to Brookfield 'learning to think critically is one of the most significant activities in adult life'.[5] So what is it?

Activity 3.1

Before reading any further, write down what you think the term 'critical thinking' means.

According to the Concise Oxford Dictionary, the word critical means 'making or involving adverse or censorious comments or judgements'.[6] It can be associated with faultfinding and carries negative overtones. Perhaps for this reason critical thinking is sometimes viewed in negative terms. People who think critically may be perceived as cynical individuals who condemn the efforts of others. It could be argued the opposite is true; critical thinking can be viewed as a positive activity. People who think critically are more likely to be aware of the diversity of values, behaviours and social structures existing around them.

An integral part of critical thinking is seeking to differentiate between assumptions and fact. An assumption according to Halpern is a 'statement for which no proof or evidence is offered'.[7] Although assumptions can be stated (explicit) or unstated (implicit), they are most often unstated or implied. Advertising provides us with frequent instances of stated and unstated assumptions. If we take the advertising of cars as an example, the explicit statement is that the car is reliable, functional and will deliver the goods. The implicit and probably more powerful message is that its owner will have high social status, and be intelligent and sexually attractive. Critical thinking involves being aware of the assumptions under which we and others behave. Such thinkers become cautious or sceptical of single solutions to problems. They become more open to new and alternative ways of looking at and behaving in the world. Critical thinking is an activity permeating all areas in our adult life and is not confined solely to learning in higher education.

Brookfield identifies four components of critical thinking.[5]

Identifying and challenging assumptions

The world in which we live is exceedingly complex and whilst containing concrete things it is not in itself a single concrete reality. Understanding of our world is inevitably shaped and influenced by our values, beliefs and attitudes. Equally the values, attitudes and beliefs of others shape our view of the world. Critical thinking involves identifying and challenging the assumptions or the 'taken-for granted' ideas, beliefs, values and behaviours of self and others. It involves asking awkward or difficult questions about habitual ways of thinking and behaving. For example critical thinkers would question the validity of the view 'workers are there to work, not to think', or decisions made by such people as 'executive directors, parents, and presidents are infallible and inviolable'.

A prime example of this, in fact, is the change in nurse education over the years. Change came about because of a challenge to the assumption that the traditional system would be suitable for a changing society.

Challenging the importance of context

Critical thinking will always be influenced by context in that thinking cannot take place within a vacuum. It is always subject to the influence of context in terms of place, time and current ideologies. An example of the influence of context can be seen by referring to the dress code of the nursing profession. Opinions regarding the accepted standard of dress and appearance of nursing staff are probably based on the norms of previous generations. Hairstyles eminently suitable in a social context may in some way be frowned upon or disapproved of in a historically conservative nursing context. The question to ask is, does an individual's hairstyle affect his or her performance as a safe and effective practising nurse?

Imagining and exploring alternatives

Critical thinkers are aware of how context shapes our habitual ways of thinking and living. They realise that many of our assumptions might be inappropriate for our lives and they are continually exploring new and alternative ways of thinking about issues or problems. As human beings we tend to find comfort in consistency in our surroundings and those things that are familiar to us. We also find similar comfort in consistent outputs from familiar processes. In other words, if we do something in a consistent way we are likely to be able to second-guess the outcome. This is acceptable if we are to take a view that nothing needs to change. However, we must ask ourselves if this is a situation in which progress will be made. If we look back through history, a number of important people spring to mind. Archimedes, Leonardo Da Vinci, Einstein, the list is endless. What is common to all of these people is their capacity to think 'out of the box'. Because things were always undertaken in a particular way or the fact that some tasks were seen as impossible, had little meaning to them. To them these seemingly great restrictions were irresistible challenges.

Reflective scepticism

Reflective scepticism ties in closely to the previously discussed components. Critical thinkers do not accept situations at face value. What becomes important to the critical thinker is not *who* says something, but *what* is said. In essence this is the basis of a philosophical approach to thinking.

Activity 3.2

Why is critical thinking so important in nursing?

Nursing is a profession most associated with 'doing' things. It has been and largely still is, a practice-based profession. However, almost all the activities nurses undertake require high-level thinking. According to Scheffer and Rubenfield thinking, feeling and doing are all essential components of nursing.[8] Thinking without doing becomes no more than an academic exercise. Doing without thinking may be dangerous, and doing and thinking without feeling is practically impossible. They defined critical thinking in nursing as '... an essential component of professional accountability and quality nursing care'. They went on to identify that critical thinkers in nursing exhibit the following habits of the mind:[8]

- confidence
- contextual perspective
- creativity
- flexibility
- inquisitiveness
- intellectual integrity
- intuition
- open-mindedness
- perseverance
- reflection.

The ability to question beyond the obvious is a major component of critical thinking. According to Brookfield critical thinking is '... at the heart of what it means to be a developed person living in a democratic society'. This ability is '... crucial to understanding our personal relationships, envisioning alternative and more productive ways of organising the workplace and becoming politically literate'.

It is important to recognise that critical thinking is not restricted to academic activity. Thayer-Bacon suggested in addition to reasoning, that critical thinkers also require 'the ability to be receptive and caring, open to others' ideas and willing to attend to them, to listen and consider other possibilities'.[9] Being a critical thinker involves more than cognitive processes such as logical reasoning; it involves recognising the assumptions underlying our beliefs and behaviours. It involves understanding how beliefs, attitudes and values influence our behaviour.

> **Activity 3.3**
>
> Before reading any further, make notes in relation to your own understanding of beliefs, attitudes and values.

Beliefs

By the time we reach adulthood we will have developed literally thousands of beliefs concerning what is true or not true about the world in which we live. A belief, according to Rokeach 'is any simple proposition, conscious or unconscious, inferred from what a person says or does'.[10] It is a descriptive thought a person holds about something. However, when someone says, 'I believe all people are equal,' for example, he or she may not be relaying their true beliefs. There are many reasons why this verbal expression may not be taken at face value. There may be compelling social or personal reasons for this, both at conscious and subconscious levels. A person may be unwilling or unable to reveal his true self to others. Although beliefs cannot be directly observed, they may, however, be inferred through the believer's actions.

Attitudes

Rokeach defines an attitude as 'a relatively enduring organisation of beliefs around an object or situation predisposing one to respond in some preferential manner'.[10] In a similar fashion to beliefs, attitudes cannot be seen; they are inferred by the actions or behaviour of an individual. Attitudes are formed as a result of direct and secondhand experience. They are the result of a lifetime of learning. Throughout life, the way in which we are raised, our contact with the rest of society, and our whole process of socialisation influences the development of our attitudes.

Attitudes have been described by Secord and Beckman as having three component parts:[11]

- a cognitive component
- an affective component
- a motor component.

The cognitive component consists of the individual's *knowledge* in relation to the attitudinal object. This cognitive component has also been described as the beliefs or ideas which the individual holds in relation to the attitudinal object. The affective part is concerned with the individual's *feelings* in relation to the object of attention. In other words, this comprises the extent to which the individual feels favourably or otherwise towards the object. The motor component refers to the *action* an individual may take. The action is the tendency or predisposition (as a result of beliefs and feelings) to behave or act in relation to the attitudinal object. To put this into context consider, for example, the student nurse who displays a seemingly negative attitude towards people with learning disabilities. The student may have a set of beliefs about such people, perhaps believing they are a burden to society. The student may also have associated feelings of disgust, despair or irritation. This belief and associated feelings may then predispose them to behave in a particular way towards such people. She may shy away from close contact or develop avoidance tactics, such as taking time off sick whilst undertaking the particular placement.

Values

The types of beliefs and attitudes people hold are indications of their values. A value is an individual's notion as to what constitutes right and wrong. Values are concerned with moral judgements to do with an individual's sense of what is desirable, good, valuable and worthwhile. To one individual, 'truth, beauty and freedom' may be top of their list, to another 'thrift, order and cleanliness'.[10] Values are deeply held and are important enough for us to maintain even in the face of pressure to change. According to Griseri '... part of being a whole, integrated person is that my values are deeply linked in with many other aspects of my personality. A change in ethics does not, cannot, happen on its own, but must inevitably affect many other elements. Hence the sheer inertia of these means that we hold tenaciously to our values. If one were not so tenacious, one might question how far their ethical views were genuinely held at all.'[12]

It is clear that attitudes, values and beliefs do not exist in isolation from each other but are inextricably linked and collectively they provide the basis for nurses' assumptions and ultimately the drive behind nurses' actions.

How do practitioners develop critical thinking?

Activity 3.4

Having considered the previous text consider for a moment those factors which are likely to influence your ability to think critically.

You will not become a critical thinker purely by reading this chapter. However, the fact that you are reading it suggests you are motivated to learn about critical thinking. First it is necessary to develop the attitude and disposition of a critical thinker. Developing the appropriate attitude and disposition is as important as developing and refining the skills. Critical thinkers are motivated and willing to exert the effort towards gathering new information; they are excited at the prospect of discovery.

Critical thinkers tend not to close down on options; more frequently they demonstrate persistence when the solution is not straightforward. They rarely give up. They are willing to take on new ideas, think in new ways, review evidence and maintain impetus until the task is complete. Critical thinkers are constantly checking for accuracy, validity and reliability of information. We may know people who, when faced with a difficult or complicated task, say 'I can't', without further thought. They are defeated from the start. They opt out of tasks which they perceive as difficult often without even beginning the thinking process. Quality thinking can be hard work. Mentally it can be as exhausting as physical exertion. The reality is that critical thinking requires hard work, diligence and persistence.

Critical thinking by its very nature requires clear, precise, purposeful thinking. Quinn suggested that critical thinkers require the ability to:[13]

- define a problem
- select relevant information for problem solving
- draw inferences from observed or supposed facts
- recognise assumptions
- formulate relevant hypotheses
- make deductions, i.e. draw conclusions from premises
- make interpretations from data
- evaluate arguments.

In essence, when considering a problem or a set of events it is essential to approach the task in a logical and ordered fashion. This helps to provide a greater degree of consistency to the way problems or issues are approached. To begin with, outline the problem or issue. When working with others, be sure that everyone has a common understanding of the problem. It is difficult to arrive at an objectively correct answer if the problem is ill defined in the first place, or if each group member has different perceptions as to what the problem is.

Finding solutions to problems is not always an easy task. A critical thinker will need a range of problem solving strategies at his or her disposal. It may be that more information is needed, or simply another perspective. The problem may be too complex, in which case consideration may be given to breaking it down into smaller, more manageable components. Another problem solving strategy that may be used involves working backwards. Instead of starting from the beginning with the problem, start from the end with the anticipated goal. This is sometimes an effective strategy to employ when there seem to be more paths leading from the goal than there are from the problem. Brainstorming is another useful way of generating options; it can be beneficial in groups or individually. It is useful to consider a whole variety of options, even outlandish ones. Sometimes it is the wild ideas that trigger solutions.

Critical thinkers can formulate ideas or a hunch (hypothesis) about problems, enabling systematic investigations to be undertaken that confirm or disprove their theories. Having acquired a wealth of information it is important to be able to do something productive with it. Critical thinkers are able to draw inferences from the facts or supposed facts. They are able to differentiate between facts, truths and assumptions and they are able to arrive at conclusions as a result of analysing and evaluating the arguments.

Consider the following exercise, which is intentionally divorced from nursing issues, allowing you to concentrate on the principles involved rather than the content.

Activity 3.5

Consider one article from a newspaper, magazine or journal and answer the following questions.

- What does the article profess to be about?
- What are the main assumptions, and are they explicit or implicit?
- What are the facts?
- Who wrote the article? Is he or she an authority on the subject? What could the author's motives be in writing the article?

Having undertaken the exercise it is important first of all to acknowledge there are no specific 'right' answers. We receive news and information from all parts of the world, in many different forms and through many different medias. Each provider of news and information will have their own reasons for such provision. It may be to do with money, to influence your point of view and ultimately to influence your judgement in some way. At the time this chapter was written, a General Election was imminent, and the media presented massive amounts of 'news'. However, it is important to consider how much of this was to inform us and how much was to influence the way we would vote. These principles apply equally to your area of work. Within critical thinking, all information must be sifted, and during this sifting you will seek to determine levels of truth or fact, identify assumptions, analyse the arguments and ultimately reach conclusions.

It is also important to consider the language used in the article you read. Was it emotive? Was it persuasive? When language is used appropriately it can clarify issues and processes. However, people frequently use language in specific ways to achieve specific results. For example, they may use persuasive words and tones, if it is their intention to sell a product or ideology. Ultimately it is their intention to manipulate how and what we think. Critical thinkers recognise such tactics and are able to respond accordingly.

Critical thinking requires the ability to use consistent and clear means of communication. Even from early childhood we all quickly become aware of the power of language and the many variations and ways in which we use language. This is apparent in the wide variety of accents, dialects and colloquial language. Whilst enhancing the richness of a local culture, a narrow or local use of language or terminology can lead to confusion and misunderstandings when applied to a wider audience. For any true critical evaluative thinking to take place it is essential that common assumptions are established and agreed, with an associated agreement as to the definition of terminology used. Take a look at the following true story that displays the ease by which we can misunderstand language and its context.

> Two elderly ladies were interviewed in Edinburgh regarding their views on tattoos. One lady expressed the opinion that they were colourful, enjoyable and provided entertainment and enjoyment for many people. The second lady disagreed vehemently, expressing a view that they were unnecessary at best, damaging at worst and somewhat vulgar. After some while the interviewer realised the first lady was referring to military tattoos. The second lady was referring to tattoos applied to the body.

Developing effective communication and interpersonal skills is essential to critical thinkers. Clear and effective communication requires thought and practice and people vary in their ability to communicate effectively. It is important to understand other people's communication and to be understood by others. Moreover, it is important to be aware of the messages conveyed by non-verbal communication. An understanding of verbal and non-verbal communication can encourage the development of trust and enables you to gain the facts required for sound and logical reasoning.

Consider the following exercise which is designed to help you to evaluate aspects of your own verbal communication skills.

Activity 3.6

Without rehearsing, tape record or video a five-minute presentation on an issue with which you are familiar. Replay the tape and listen to what you have said with reference to the following questions.

- Was the overall purpose of the talk clear?
- Did you get the main points across?

- Did the talk develop in a logical manner?
- Was your voice strong and confident or was it too quiet and hesitant?
- Did you sound as if you knew what you were talking about?

Principles of effective communication apply to verbal, written and electronic communication. Comprehensive hand-over sessions, adequate referral information and legible and unambiguous patient notes is, without doubt, of paramount importance. The ability to organise your thoughts and views in written form is as important as being able to provide a coherent verbal account. The written presentation of ideas facilitates the application of critical thinking principles. For example, before putting pen to paper (or fingers to keyboard) you will need to determine an organised approach to the work. You will need to make a decision regarding what is relevant and what is superfluous and in the process of clarifying your own thoughts you will, no doubt, consider other perspectives in relation to the subject. Many of the principles outlined in the previous section apply to writing skills. The style and organisation of written work will depend on the purpose of the account. However, it is worth remembering that any documentation that cannot be read and/or interpreted is of little value in terms of communication.

Facilitating critical thinking in others

Activity 3.7

How can you assist the development of critical thinking skills in students?

Both nurses and student nurses come into the profession with a variety of thinking skills. According to Rubenfield and Scheffer '... enhancing thinking is a deliberate act that can be taught and learned'. However, it is important to *nurture* the development of such skills. Brookfield identified a number of 'positive approaches' that can be used to facilitate the development of critical thinking in others.[5]

Affirm critical thinkers' self-worth

Forcing students to critically analyse their assumptions influencing how they live and think may serve to alienate and intimidate them, engendering a resistance to the entire process. A skilled mentor will awaken, encourage and nurture the student without making them feel either threatened or patronised. The mentor must balance between respecting the integrity of the student as well as at the same time asking sufficiently challenging questions which prompt them to examine their assumptions. Challenging other peoples' assumptions requires practice and skill. Challenge should always be offered in a supportive manner and should not degenerate into an attack on the other person.

Activity 3.8

Ask a student to discuss his or her attitude towards people who smoke, despite the harmful effects to their health.
Does the student believe it would be acceptable to withhold any required treatment if the individual could not guarantee to give up?

What effect might you have on the student if you are confrontational in asking them to defend their views?

Show that you support critical thinkers' efforts

Students require time, encouragement and support, balanced with the necessary degree of challenge, to stimulate the development of their critical thinking skills. In addition to celebrating students' success, mentors need to support the student in such a way that allows them to 'risk failure without feeling that in doing so they have actually failed'.

Activity 3.9

Students may meet ethical dilemmas without having had the opportunity to prepare for them.
How can you encourage them to articulate and develop their ideas?

Reflect and mirror critical thinkers' ideas and actions

It is difficult for individuals to view their own taken-for-granted ideas, values, attitudes and assumptions and to interpret personal actions and behaviours in an objective way. However, the mentor can use a technique known as 'mirroring' to 'reflect' back an individual's attitudes, motivations and justifications, helping students to explore and become more aware of how their behaviours and attitudes may be perceived by others.

Activity 3.10

How can you help students to become more aware of their own beliefs and attitudes?

Motivate people to think critically and listen attentively to critical thinkers

Motivation influences learning and this is strongly affected by the student's degree of interest. Whilst the motivation for learning ultimately lies with the student, mentors can be a catalyst by helping them to realise ideas they may have only considered tentatively in the past. In addition to this it is also important to know when to provide support. This involves approving, confirming or validating the student's experience; listening to their views and respecting and valuing their contributions.

Regularly evaluate progress

Of equal importance is the need for effective evaluation of progress. As students develop it is very easy to forget where they started from; critical thinking becomes 'a way of life' and students may adopt the view that they have always thought in this way. They should be encouraged to consider their starting point and where their critical thinking has taken them. In this way, we provide opportunities for students to understand their critical thinking skills, gain insights into their own behaviour patterns and those of others. They are also able to make informed judgement on the effectiveness and consequences of their actions. Alongside this is the need to alert individuals to the potential risks associated with the consequences of challenging established values and practices. Part of the skill of critical thinking is developing an understanding (which is almost intuitive) as to when would be the 'right' time and place to pose such a challenge. When would it have most impact? How should the challenge be posed? Should it be posed at all? Put simply, will this challenge result in the desired outcome or will it result in a negative outcome?

Help critical thinkers to create networks

Students are often involved in working together in group tasks and projects, indeed social learning of this nature is frequently associated with successful learning.[14] Since identifying and challenging assumptions brings with it many aspects of threat and risk taking, the safety and security of group working and problem solving can yield benefits. As a mentor responsible for students in your clinical area, you could develop opportunities for group work by asking students to prepare a discussion on the pros and cons of electroconvulsive therapy or the withholding of treatment for a patient who is likely to die regardless of intervention. Projects of this nature will help students to feel supported by their peers and will also help to develop useful networks.

Be critical teachers

Inherent within the role of mentor is a specific teaching role. As critical teachers, mentors can create a climate for critical thinking by questioning assumptions, promoting inquiry, taking risks and experimenting with new ideas during their teaching. They can create a learning climate where it is safe to experiment, take risks and make mistakes, provided a reasonable process was followed.

Make people aware of how they learn critical thinking

Helping people to understand their personal styles and patterns of learning is one of the most important aspects of aiding the development of critical thinking. Helping students to gain insight and to understand what it is that motivates them, how they integrate new ideas and experience, and how they learn new information, is crucial to the development of critical thinking.

Model critical thinking

Since it has been acknowledged for some time that a significant amount of learning will take place as a result of 'role modelling', it is essential that mentors model critical thinking in their practice.[15] Students are likely to learn the process by observing the clarity, consistency and logic demonstrated by their mentor.

The previous section provides a useful checklist which will help you to support students in the development of their thinking. In addition to this there are a variety of learning strategies which may be employed by mentors and which can facilitate the development of critical thinking in students. The most effective learning strategies will have relevance to the student and relate to their practice. You may, for example, give students a task which involves the use of problem solving skills, such as asking them to produce a report which comments on the care received by an individual patient. In doing this you are asking students to think critically. You are asking them to identify assumptions, distinguish between relevant and irrelevant information, recognise inconsistencies, and identify patterns and missing information. You are asking them to draw conclusions based on evidence. All of these skills are component parts of the skill of critical thinking.

Conclusion

The importance of the development of critical thinking in pre-registration programmes has been confirmed within *Fitness for Practice*.[1] The need to encourage and develop creative, critical thinkers who can respond to the rapidly changing healthcare environment is considered to be crucial. The role of mentors in students' development of this skill is evident. If it is accepted that a significant amount of student learning occurs as a result of their observations of good role models, it follows that mentors adopting a critical thinking approach in their practice will facilitate the development of critical thinking in students. In addition, mentors need to nurture the development of critical thinking in students, taking time to explore their values, attitudes and beliefs, helping them to understand how these influence or impinge on their practice.

The acquisition of critical thinking has been portrayed as something of a journey, complex and tortuous at times, but well worth the effort. However, it should be acknowledged that whilst there is the potential for developing critical thinking in many situations, ultimately it is up to the student to take the initiative and make a commitment to taking the process forward.

References

1 UKCC (1999) *Fitness for Practice*. UKCC, London.

2 UKCC (2000) *Requirements for Pre-Registration Nursing Programmes*. UKCC, London.

3 Saxton J and Ashworth P (1990) On competence. *Journal of Higher Education*. **14**: 1–24.

4 Swendsen Boss L (1985) Teaching for Clinical Competence. *Nurse Educator*. **10**: 8–12.

5 Brookfield SD (1987) *Developing Critical Thinkers: challenging adults to explore alternative ways of thinking and acting*. Open University Press, Buckingham.

6 Allen RE (1990) *Concise Oxford Dictionary of Current English* (8e). Clarendon Press, Oxford.

7 Halpern DF (1997) *Critical Thinking Across the Curriculum: a brief edition of thought and knowledge*. Lawrence Erlbaum Associates, London, p. 102.

8   Scheffer BK and Rubenfeld MG (1999) *Critical Thinking in Nursing: an interactive approach* (2e). Lippincott, Philadelphia, p. 376.

9   Thayer-Bacon BJ (1993) Caring and its relationship to critical thinking. *Educational Theory.* **43**: 323–40.

10 Rokeach M (1972) *Beliefs, Attitudes and Values.* Jossey-Bass, London.

11 Secord PF and Backman CW (1964) *Social Psychology.* McGraw-Hill, New York.

12 Griseri P (1998) *Managing Values: ethical change in organisations.* Macmillan, London, p. 115–16.

13 Quinn FM (1997) *The Principles and Practice of Nurse Education.* Stanley Thornes, Cheltenham, p. 50.

14 Jarvis P (1987) *Learning in the Social Context.* Croom Helm, London.

15 Ogier ME (1989) *Working and Learning: the learning environment in clinical nursing.* Scutari, London.

CHAPTER FOUR

How are they doing?
Assessing your students

Chapter overview

- Introduction
- Definition and principles of assessment
- Types of assessment
- Determining learning needs
- Reviewing progress
- Judging achievement
- Objectivity of assessment
- Partnership in assessment
- A new framework for preparation of mentors and teachers
- Conclusion

Introduction

The primary aim of pre-registration programmes is 'to ensure that students are prepared to practise safely and effectively, to such an extent that the protection of the public is assured'.[1] To ensure this aim is achieved, pre-registration education programmes must be dynamic and able to respond to the many complexities of changing practice. The new requirements for pre-registration programmes have been re-focused on an outcome-based competency framework. It is a fundamental principle of the new programmes that they should be practice-centred and directed towards the achievement of professional competence.[2] These developments have implications for the way in which students are assessed both now and in the future.

In considering assessment, it is important to acknowledge the diversity of students in terms of life experience and their previous experiences of traditional examination format. Any assessment method used, whilst ensuring the proper preparation of the student, must also have the capacity to bring out their best performance. In doing so, the likelihood is increased that students will develop a positive and willing approach to lifelong learning. The contribution that clinical staff make to this process is vital. However, they require the appropriate knowledge, skills and values in order to prepare students for this dynamic world of healthcare and as such will have their own steep learning curve.

So far in this book we have explored ways in which confidence can be developed in teaching. We are now moving on to consider assessment, an essential component of the learning process. A number of fundamental principles are important for the successful assessment of students in practice. The purpose of this chapter is to discuss and explore these further.

Definition and principles of assessment

Activity 4.1

Before reading any further, make notes on what you consider to be the purpose of assessing students.

Assessment is a way in which we determine the extent to which learning has taken place. In educational terms, the main functions of assessment are:

- to establish a baseline for future development; this relates to the initial assessment, and is undertaken to establish the students' future learning needs. It is an essential prerequisite to the effective planning of future teaching
- to measure current performance; in this context assessment is seen as a process by which a student's level of competence, achievement or performance is assessed.

Rowntree identifies six reasons for assessing students:[3]

- to select for educational courses or careers
- to maintain standards
- to motivate students
- to give feedback to students
- to give feedback to teachers
- to prepare students for life (in the sense of getting them used to working in a world where their performance will be subject to scrutiny).

The range and types of assessment that can be used vary considerably and the purposes of such assessments are equally varied. However, Quinn suggests whichever type of assessment is used it should conform to the following basic aims:[4]

- to assess student performance in relation to the aims of the particular programme in question
- to be regarded as an integral component of the teaching and learning process, and not simply as a means of measuring attainment
- to encourage the student to undertake self-assessment and reflection on their learning.

To be able to assess accurately and effectively, mentors need to be familiar with the:

- overall aims of the student's programme
- outcomes for entry to the branch programme (*see* Appendix)
- competencies for entry to the register (*see* Appendix)
- specific outcomes and competencies which students should achieve whilst on placement
- expected level of achievement in relation to the identified outcomes and competencies.

Types of assessment

Formative and summative assessment

Before we examine the main types of assessment with which you will need to be familiar, give some thought to the following exercise.

> ## Activity 4.2
>
> In relation to assessment, what do you think the following terms mean?
>
> - Formative
> - Summative
> - Continuous
> - Episodic

Assessment is either formative or summative. Formative assessment refers to the process of ascertaining the student's progress *during* a period of study. Normally there is no mark or grade attached to this work and it does not directly affect final end-of-course grades. However, used appropriately, formative work is a valuable way for the student to obtain feedback on performance or progress whilst working towards the summative assessments. An example of this in clinical practice may be the presentation of the main elements of a care study to the care team. Constructive feedback from the team provides the student with the opportunity of strengthening any weak elements of the care study both in practice and in written form. The student is then able to produce a final piece of work that is submitted as part of the summative assessment at the *end* of a course or unit of study.

Summative assessment refers to the formal assessment of learning that has taken place and counts towards the overall mark at the end of the period of study. You can see that the formative work allows students to 'practise' without the stress of being formally graded for their efforts.

> ## Activity 4.3
>
> It could be argued that students should be graded for their efforts, even at the formative stage.
> How does this relate to the notion of motivation, discussed in Chapter 2.

Continuous assessment

In recent years there has been a trend to continuous assessment perhaps reflecting the complexities of the learning process and the nature of nursing itself. The English National Board (ENB) defined continuous assessment as 'a planned series of progressively updated measurements of student achievement and progress'.[5] It is an ongoing process *throughout* the course, and involves sampling a student's practice on a continuous basis. As an assessment method it has a number of advantages over episodic forms of assessment (examinations taken at specific times or occasions during the educational programme); it takes into account the probability that students may have one-off bad days and ensures that their performance is assessed in real-life situations.

The disadvantages are that some students feel under constant pressure to achieve and some students may be reluctant to ask questions to avoid bringing attention to what they perceive as their lack of ability. In the college or university setting, continuous assessment is generally focused on assessing all of the student's coursework, for example, essays, care studies, examinations, projects and presentations. As a method of assessment it allows the student and lecturer to build up a complete profile of the student's achievements throughout the course.

Formal and informal

Formal assessment usually refers to a range of assessments undertaken during a course of study. Written examinations, essays, care studies and module or unit assessments are all examples of formal assessments. Informal assessment on the other hand is frequently undertaken on a day-to-day basis by the lecturer or the mentor. It is unobtrusive in nature and is concerned with the day-to-day work and learning of the student. Information is gathered from informal contact or interviews with the student. Essentially this information provides additional evidence to the mentor or the lecturer and assists them in reaching a reasoned judgement regarding the student's performance.

Portfolio

A portfolio in itself is not a method of assessment, it is a collection of materials that may include the individual's reflections, profiles, project work and results of peer and self-assessments. At its simplest level Redman suggests that a portfolio is simply a tangible record of what someone has done.[6] It has been described as a private collection of evidence which demonstrates the continuing acquisition of skills, knowledge, attitudes, understanding and achievement. It is both retrospective and prospective, as well as reflecting the current stage of development of the individual.[7]

Activity 4.4

What are the benefits of portfolios to the student and the mentor?

Portfolios can be used to achieve greater congruence between what is learned in the classroom and on practice placements. The keeping of portfolios for pre-registration nursing students is a requirement of the ENB[8] and was re-emphasised in *Fitness for Practice*[1] which states that 'portfolios should demonstrate a student's fitness for practice and provide evidence of rational decision-making and clinical judgement'. The new preparation for practice identifies four domains:

- professional and ethical practice
- care delivery
- care management
- personal and professional development.

The student is required to demonstrate competency in each of these domains (*see* Appendix). The domain of personal and professional development makes explicit the requirement for individual learning through the development of a portfolio of practice.[2] Students, therefore, must be encouraged to develop a cumulative portfolio incorporating formal and informal learning which can then be used to inform the assessment process in both theory and practice. Portfolios require regular review and updating in order to help students to:

- understand how they learn
- organise and plan their own learning
- provide evidence of what they have achieved to date
- develop self-assessment skills
- focus on personal and professional experiences

- develop skills of reflection
- develop the skills necessary for maintaining a portfolio
- prepare for future employment.

A typical student portfolio may contain any or all of the following (those areas identified in italics relate to the ENB requirements and must be included in the portfolio):[8]

- curriculum vitae
- details of any course/experiences
- *cumulative information about the student's achievement of outcomes and learning through reflection, demonstrating the interrelationship of theory and practice*
- reflective diary/critical incidents
- transcript of training
- *the outcomes of assessment of both theory and practice*
- *issues raised in discussion including causes for concern between the mentor, the student and the personal/named lecturer*
- *an action plan or learning contract agreed between the mentor, the student and the personal tutor/named lecturer*
- *key issues from the student's experience which will inform the preparation for subsequent experience*
- placement/clinical assessments
- assignments
- details of seminar presentations
- feedback from assignments/clinical experience.

In essence the development of a portfolio by the student is crucial to successfully achieving qualified status. Throughout the duration of the programme students collect evidence of their learning (*see* Box 4.1) which shows they have achieved the UKCC outcomes and competencies (*see* Appendix). Table 4.1 provides an example of a developmental learning plan which may be used to collect such evidence.

Some aspects of the student's practice may not be demonstrated by performance alone. In these circumstances questioning may be used to probe underpinning knowledge in relation to specific aspects of care provision. Where evidence is of a verbal nature, it can be used to inform the mentor's judgement of the student's progress during the placement. Later it can be incorporated into subsequent written assessments compiled by the mentor.

Box 4.1 Evidence collected by the student for the development of a portfolio

Placement/practice activities
This may take the form of evidence in relation to the student's:

- evidence of professional experiences
- contribution to patient care, situations, procedures
- contribution to team meetings, personal tutorials
- learning contracts
- assessment of practice forms
- involvement in research projects.

University/college-based activities
This may take the form of evidence in relation to the student's:

- assignments/projects/ seminar work
- other educational accomplishments
- relevant certificates/courses of study.

Third party testimony
This may take the form of:

- written and verbal feedback from other professionals, patients and their families or clinical mentors.

Personal accounts
This may take the form of:

- written and verbal account of work
- personal reflections of learning and work activities
- personal achievements.

Direct observation and questioning
This may take the form of:

- observation of student's work/practice by the mentor/other professionals/ team members
- questioning and discussion between mentor and the student.

Self and peer assessment

Activity 4.5

What is self-assessment and how can mentors encourage self-assessment in students?

Table 4.1   A developmental learning plan (Liverpool John Moores University)[9]

Learning goals	Learning resources/strategies	Evidence of achievement and evaluation learning goals
What will I know or be able to do after completion of placement?	What resources will I need and how will I organise my actions?	By demonstrating progress towards goal accomplishment which can be assessed via mentor, self, client or peer.
• To measure and record vital signs (blood pressure, pulse, temperature, respiration) accurately • To measure fluid input/output and chart findings accurately • To measure height and weight and record results appropriately • To record peak flow readings and chart results accurately	• Observing other practitioners undertaking and recording observations • Supervised practice of observations • Reference to ward policies and procedures	• Will have successfully completed elements of the skills inventory related to the measurement and recording of results • Have an appreciation of the importance of accurate documentation of results relating to care
• To have an understanding of the function of the ward-based information technology systems	• Observe ward staff using the applications in the clinical environment • Refer to the Data Protection Act • Telephone communication	• To be able to discuss the use of the applications in the clinical areas • To discuss the consequences of the inappropriate use of such systems • To answer the telephone appropriately
• To be able to attend to patients' hygiene and toileting needs in response to the individual's wants/ preferences • Maintain standards acceptable to patients, considering the maintenance of privacy, dignity, comfort and safety	• Participate in a variety of situations to ensure the maintenance of hygiene/toileting and personal care needs are appropriately met (e.g. bed-bathing, assisted washes at the bedside, appropriate use of commode)	• To have observed and participated in a range of methods of assisting patients to maintain hygiene/toileting needs • Will have successfully completed elements of the skills inventory relating to personal care

In self-assessment, students are actively encouraged to evaluate their own performance. This may be accomplished through a written piece of work, perhaps a reflective account of their performance in practice, or it may be an oral account. The activity centres around the student, encouraging them to be critical of their strengths and weaknesses. It is a useful strategy to employ when assessing students in clinical practice and provides an excellent basis on which to give students feedback on their progress or performance. When assessing their performance, students can sometimes focus on the most negative or weakest aspect of their practice. Whilst this gives the mentor an opportunity to suggest ways of rectifying the difficulty, it is important to provide a balance by helping the student to identify positive elements within their practice.

Peer assessment is another student-centred method of assessment and can be used by two or more students, preferably working in small groups. It is the assessment of a student by his or her fellow students.

Activity 4.6

What are the benefits of peer assessment?

Peer assessment provides students with the opportunity to learn from the feedback of colleagues, and it also provides a sound foundation for any future role which involves critically appraising the work or performance of others. Whilst peer assessment can be very effective, it should be used with caution if the work is to be awarded a mark which contributes to the final grade. Whilst students should be given the opportunity for peer assessment, mentors are not absolved of responsibility within the process and need to maintain at least a peripheral involvement. It is possible for 'over-enthusiastic' students to collude in giving each other high marks which may not relate directly to their performance.

Determining learning needs

Activity 4.7

How can the mentor prepare for a student who is about to start a placement?

Students require competent, confident mentors in practice. Being prepared for the student will increase your level of confidence. Ask yourself the following questions *before* the student arrives.

- Do you know the student's name?
- How long is this planned experience?
- What are the learning outcomes determined by the curriculum and what is their relationship to this placement?
- Do you know what stage of the course the student has reached?
- What is the overall philosophy of the course?
- How many hours will the student be working? Is he or she entitled to any additional study time whilst on placement in your clinical or practice area?
- Is the student expected to complete any coursework whilst on this placement?
- If the answer to the above question is yes, what does this work consist of, what are the deadlines, what are the marking criteria?
- How can you help?

You can find out the answers to some of these questions by contacting the designated link teacher or lecturer or the course leader at the college or university. Having this information to hand when the student arrives not only demonstrates commitment, motivation and professionalism on your part, it also helps you to anticipate some of the learning needs of the student before they arrive for the first interview. Ideally the mentor should meet with the student on the first day of the placement in order to introduce the student to other members of the care team, to orient the student to the placement and outline health and safety procedures within the unit. It is useful to plan this meeting in advance, arranging for a suitable room to be made available where there is less chance of distractions or interruptions.

Activity 4.8

Make a list of the main issues that need to be addressed at the initial interview.

It is likely that in addition to the specific learning outcomes students must achieve during practice placements, they may also have additional, personal goals to achieve. It is useful at this early stage to establish a mutual plan of action in relation to the organisation of the learning experience and the mechanisms for assessing progress. During the interview the mentor can use the previously gained information to tease out specific individual learning needs and discuss any concerns or anxieties the student may have. Specific dates should be identified and arrangements made to meet with students mid-way through and towards the end of the placement experience. A useful way of organising this initial meeting and subsequent meetings is through the use of a learning agreement. Whilst not totally binding, it is a way of identifying achievable, realistic and measurable learning outcomes.

Reviewing progress

Activity 4.9

How can the mentor prepare for an interim progress assessment?

In preparation for the mid-way interview, the mentor may gain feedback from other members of the care team, in relation to the student's performance and progress. Students may be requested to reflect on their experiences so far and assess the extent to which identified practice competencies have been met. They will need time to undertake this activity and it would, therefore, be advisable to discuss these expectations during the initial interview.

The main purpose of the mid-way interview is to discuss the student's progress and performance so far, to identify strengths, achievements, weaknesses and areas requiring further development. At this stage both mentor and student should have a clear idea of whether the student is achieving the required level of performance. If a student is failing, it is important to identify precisely where he or she is experiencing difficulties as soon as possible. A decision must be made as to whether it is appropriate to involve the link teacher or the student's personal tutor at this stage. The necessity for this will depend on the nature of the problem and the ability of the mentor and student to overcome the difficulty. The development of an action plan for the remainder of the placement should provide the student with the opportunity to rectify the problem. It may also be necessary to arrange more frequent meetings between the mentor and the student in order to monitor progress effectively. As with the initial interview, an accurate written account of these meetings must be retained by both the mentor and the student.

Judging achievement

Activity 4.10

How can a mentor prepare for a student's final assessment?

At the end of the practice experience the mentor makes a judgement in relation to the student's performance and achievement of competence. In order to make this judgement, mentors need to:

Observe: The mentor should be particularly observant when working with students. Observations need not be formal, but the role of a mentor is to assess, therefore observation of the student in practice is crucial.

Listen: Whilst the practice of asking other people to comment on the student's performance may be of some value, there is no doubt that other people will come into contact with the student during the course of their practice. Patients, other professionals and colleagues may express a view in relation to the student's practice. This type of information may be subjective and there is great reliance on the skills of the mentor to decipher the relevance and relative importance of this information. It is important to listen to what the student has to say about their experiences and their learning so far.

Discuss: Any opportunity to discuss observations and feedback with the student should not be missed, including the student's own reflections on practice they have observed. Together they should form part of the diagnostic process and should be a continuous element of teaching and learning.

Decide: Based on the mentor's contact and discussions with the student, observations and feedback from the rest of the team, other colleagues and patients where appropriate, the mentor must decide whether the student has achieved the required level of competence. (Adapted from Jarvis and Gibson.[10])

In most cases the placement is a success and students are awarded a pass and move on to the next placement. However, in a small number of situations, students fail to reach the required level. The task of failing students is, without doubt, an onerous one. In such a situation the earlier work with the student should have made the task a little easier as the student will be aware of the mentor's standards and concerns and also of any self-assessment which might have been made. The decision to fail the student in such circumstances may not come as a surprise to the student. It is likely in such circumstances that the link teacher or the personal tutor will also be part of the process. By following the guidance provided within this section, the decision-making process is one shared by the student, the mentor, colleagues who have worked with the student and the link teacher or personal tutor. Taken in this context, the final decision is likely to be fair and well balanced, although well documented records are always essential to support any recommendation. Such documentation will be called upon in the event of a student appeal against the decision.

Objectivity of assessment

Activity 4.11

How can the mentor ensure that personal feelings towards the student do not detrimentally influence the assessment?

There are a number of issues that should be considered in relation to the objectivity of an assessment. For example, if an assessment is undertaken in relation to a patient or client, the information should provide a clear and factual picture of the patient or client. In this respect, assessment of student performance is the same. Accurate assessment requires care, time and effort if it is to be objective. Mentors should not allow their personal likes or dislikes to influence assessment. When this happens it is known as the 'halo or horn' effect. The halo effect occurs when a mentor is influenced by the positive characteristics of a student. If the mentor has a positive impression of the student, for example if the student is always polite, smartly dressed and punctual, the mentor may rate the student highly, tending to ignore poor aspects of their performance.[11] The horn effect occurs if a mentor sees unfavourable characteristics in the student, for example if the mentor is unduly influenced by previous negative assessments of the student or as a result of non-conformity on the part of the student.

Some mentors give every student an average mark irrespective of performance. This is known as *central tendency error*. Other mentors give students higher marks than are warranted, and this is referred to as *error of leniency*. A range of factors including the mentor's past experience, level of motivation, personality, beliefs, values and prejudices have an influence on assessment. How far the mentor can depend on the accuracy of their assessment will depend not only on the extent to which they have been influenced by these factors, but also on the extent to which they are aware of their own prejudices.

Activity 4.12

Think about a particular student that you recently supervised. What personal attributes did you particularly like or dislike about the student? Now consider to what extent these attributes influenced your judgement of the student's performance.

The accuracy of the assessment is also affected by four cardinal criteria:

- reliability
- validity
- discrimination
- practicality.

Irrespective of the type of assessment used, it should always be examined critically to assess to what extent it meets these criteria.

Reliability

Reliability refers to the consistency with which a test measures what it is designed to measure. It refers to the extent to which the results would be the same if the test were reapplied at a different time to the same student. A reliable test is one in which a student would gain a similar result if they completed the test on more than one occasion. Of course it should be recognised that there are a number of variables *outside* the test situation that could have a bearing on the likelihood of this happening, apart from the reliability of the test. The student's state of health, anxiety levels, home circumstances or environmental conditions surrounding the test may all have an impact on the likelihood of the student achieving the same results on more than one occasion. Equally if you as a mentor are not feeling well or not performing properly, you should realise that this may also have an impact on the assessment.

Validity

Validity is the extent to which the test or assessment measures what it is designed to measure. To put this into context, think back to the early intelligence tests. For many years it was thought that intelligence quotient (IQ) tests measured the intellectual ability of children. It was later recognised that IQ tests were more a measure of testing pupils' understanding of the English language. IQ tests did not fully measure what they were designed to measure, and they therefore lacked validity.[12] The measurement of validity tells us to what degree any test or assessment measures or describes what it is supposed to.

If an assessment method is unreliable, then it also lacks validity. However, a reliable assessment method is not necessarily valid. It could produce the same or similar responses on all occasions, but fail to measure what it is supposed to measure. This may seem relatively straightforward. However, measuring the extent of validity can become complex, particularly when considering some of the subdivisions of validity.

Face validity

This is concerned with the extent to which a particular assessment tool seems, to an experienced practitioner, to be able to achieve its stated aim. Consider the following example. A member of your staff has designed a written assessment to measure the student's ability to take a patient's blood pressure. The written assessment may ask all the right questions but can it actually measure the student's ability to take a blood pressure?

The answer is no. Taking blood pressure requires skill on the part of the student as well as knowledge. The written assessment can determine the knowledge, however it is unable to assess the skill component of the task. Without testing the tool, it is easy to see that it lacks face validity.

Content validity

This relates specifically to *what* is being addressed. For example, the assessment strategy of a programme of education should adequately sample the content of the syllabus. If it succeeds in doing this, it is able to demonstrate content validity.

Predictive validity

This indicates the extent to which any test predicts the future performance or behaviour of the student. As a general rule, the more infrequent the assessment, the less likely the assessment is able to predict the performance or behaviour of the individual. As discussed earlier in this chapter, courses leading to a qualification in nursing are now assessed continuously. This is to increase the *predictive validity* of the assessment process.

Discrimination

Discrimination relates to whether a test discriminates between those who know the answers and those who do not. A test is said to discriminate when it successfully identifies those who perform correctly and those who do not. If a test fails to discriminate between those who do and those who do not, then it has no purpose. Consider for example a group of students undertaking a first aid examination. Those students who are unable to demonstrate the appropriate knowledge and skills will fail and those who demonstrate proficiency will pass.

Practicality

An assessment or test should be practical in terms of time and resources. The practicality or the 'user friendliness' of an assessment tool can have implications for its subsequent reliability. If the assessment is a lengthy, complicated and time-consuming process, the motivation to complete the assessment may dwindle or disappear altogether.

Partnership in assessment

The ENB and Department of Health (DoH) highlight the need for robust partnerships between education and service providers.[13] This is crucial in helping to ensure students gain meaningful experiences where practice outcomes and competencies can be effectively met. It is also important to the continued professional development of clinical staff and staff within the education sector.

Students will be supported by a range of professional and academic staff during the programme. They will be allocated a *personal tutor* who is able to advise, support and facilitate learning. The role of the personal tutor has been described as assisting students to relate theory to practice;[14] smoothing the path for the students in a situation of constant change in the delivery of education and healthcare,[15] and providing academic and personal support.[16] Box 4.2 identifies the role of the personal tutor within the new programme of preparation at Liverpool John Moores University.[17]

Students will also be allocated a *mentor* who assumes responsibility for the student's learning in the practice setting. The mentor is responsible for the quality of learning, and the assessment of competencies. According to the ENB and the DoH, mentors have a responsibility to:[18]

- facilitate student learning across pre- and post-registration programmes
- supervise, support and guide students in practice in institutional and non-institutional settings
- implement approved assessment procedures.

Each practice placement is also likely to have a named *link teacher*. In this role nurse teachers or lecturers are employed and accountable to the education sector, but are expected to link with clinical practice with a view to:[19]

- supporting, guiding and facilitating students' learning
- carrying out educational audits and monitoring the clinical learning environment

- assisting qualified staff with update sessions on continuous assessment and learning contracts
- participating in joint school or clinical meetings
- spending more time working alongside students in practice.

Box 4.2   Role of the personal tutor

1   To meet and assist students in the identification of their individual learning needs.
2   To support students in the achievement of intended learning outcomes.
3   To monitor the total learning experience of individual students, including student attendance and progression.
4   To provide feedback and guidance to students on their performance in both academic and clinical coursework.
5   To provide the student with the opportunity to discuss the development of their professional portfolio.
6   To identify the special needs of students to ensure that those students are supported.
7   To maintain a record of all meetings with the student and compile a yearly report on student progress.
8   To advise the programme leader, academic centre manager or assistant director of any students who are failing to achieve, either academically or clinically.

The role of *practice educator* is a relatively new role. Practice educators play a key role in the support and supervision of pre- and post-registration students. In partnership with mentors, lecturers, nurse and other healthcare consultants, practice educators co-ordinate students' experiences and assessment of learning in practice.

In order to produce a competent practitioner, there must be effective collaboration and negotiation between the mentor, the teacher (link teacher or personal tutor) and the student.[20–22] The student requires a mentor who is readily available, clinically competent and understands the key functions of their area of practice. He or she needs a teacher who is knowledgeable about the learning needs of the student and is in a position to ensure that these are effectively met.

New framework for preparation of mentors and teachers

From September 2001 the ENB approved new mentor and teacher preparation programmes which replace the ENB 997/998 Teaching and Assessing in Clinical Practice and Community Practice Teacher programmes. All nursing, midwifery and health visiting teacher preparation will be organised within a new framework (Box 4.3).

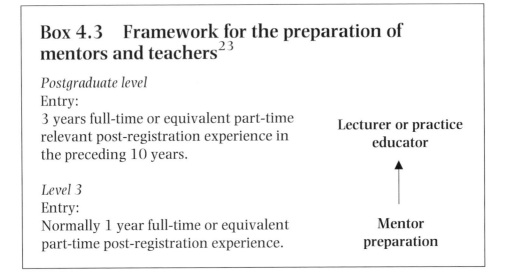

Box 4.3   Framework for the preparation of mentors and teachers[23]

Postgraduate level
Entry:
3 years full-time or equivalent part-time relevant post-registration experience in the preceding 10 years.

Lecturer or practice educator

Level 3
Entry:
Normally 1 year full-time or equivalent part-time post-registration experience.

Mentor preparation

Whilst practitioners can enter the framework at any level, it is anticipated that many practitioners will want to complete the mentorship preparation programme at an early stage in their career. Practitioners will gain credit for that part of the teaching programme and continue their development at postgraduate level at a later stage in their career. Practitioners who have current registration with the UKCC, additional professional and academic qualifications and experience applicable to the context of care delivery will be eligible for the programme. In addition to this they will also have completed at least 12 months' full-time (or equivalent part-time) experience.

In order to facilitate the development of critical analytical skills, communication and decision-making skills, the new mentor preparation programme will be delivered at a minimum of academic Level 3. The ENB and DoH state programmes of preparation should:[23]

- be developed in partnership with education and service colleagues
- be multiprofessional wherever possible
- use flexible modes of delivery, including open, distance and electronic learning.

Whilst nurses, midwives and health visitors holding the ENB 997/998 or the Community Practice Teacher qualification will not be expected to undertake the new preparation in order to act as mentors, it is anticipated that the new requirements will assist practitioners in the identification of continuing professional development needs.

The UKCC have produced eight advisory standards for the preparation of mentors which are listed in Box 4.4.[24]

Box 4.4   Advisory standards for the preparation of mentors[24]

Section 2 of the advisory standards highlights the importance of eight key areas.

1 **Communication and working relationships including**:
   - the development of effective relationships based on mutual trust and respect
   - an understanding of how students integrate into practice settings and assisting with this process
   - the provision of ongoing constructive support for students.
2 **Facilitation of learning in order to**:
   - demonstrate sufficient knowledge of the student's programme to identify current learning needs
   - demonstrate strategies which will assist with the integration of learning from practice and education settings
   - create and develop opportunities for students to identify and undertake experiences to meet their learning needs.
3 **Assessment in order to**:
   - demonstrate effective relationships with patients and clients
   - contribute to the development of an environment in which effective practice is fostered, implemented, evaluated and disseminated
   - assess and manage clinical developments to ensure safe and effective care.

4 **Role modelling in order to:**
  - demonstrate effective relationships with patients and clients
  - contribute to the development of an environment in which effective practice is fostered, implemented, evaluated and disseminated
  - assess and manage clinical developments to ensure safe and effective care.
5 **Creating an environment for learning in order to:**
  - ensure effective learning experiences and the opportunity to achieve learning
  - ensure outcomes for students by contributing to the development and maintenance of a learning environment
  - implement strategies for quality assurance and quality audit.
6 **Improving practice in order to:**
  - contribute to the creation of an environment in which change can be initiated and supported.
7 **A knowledge base in order to:**
  - identify, apply and disseminate research findings within the area of practice.
8 **Course developments which:**
  - contribute to the development and/or review of courses.

The framework provides the opportunity for further professional development throughout the career of the practitioner. Practitioners can follow one of two pathways. Lecturer programmes are aimed at preparing appropriately qualified and experienced practitioners for a role in the higher education environment, whilst practice educator programmes are aimed at preparing appropriately qualified and experienced practitioners for a role within the practice setting. Both roles have equal standing within the framework and individuals will be able to move between the role of lecturer and practice educator. There are similarities between the two programmes. Both programmes involve study at postgraduate level and the basic entry requirements are the same. Individuals should have:[23]

- an entry on an appropriate part(s) of the UKCC register (parts 1, 3, 5, 8, 10, 11, 12, 13, 14 or 15)
- completed a minimum of three years' full-time experience (or equivalent part-time experience) in relevant professional practice during the last 10 years

- acquired additional professional knowledge which must be relevant to the intended area of teaching or practice and at no less than first degree level
- three years' full-time experience (or equivalent part-time experience) in relevant professional practice in areas where students were gaining practice experience.

The theoretical underpinning of both courses of preparation is similar, although the emphasis of teaching practice undertaken within each programme is naturally focused to higher education in the case of the lecturer programme and practice in the case of the practice educator programme. Lecturer programmes of preparation equip practitioners with the necessary skills and knowledge to work as members of a teaching team within a higher education setting. Responsibilities include ensuring that learning experiences and assessment strategies enable students to meet identified learning outcomes in both education and practice settings. Practice educator programmes equip practitioners for a role within the practice setting enabling them to provide support to mentors and other practitioners contributing to the student's learning experience. On qualification, an adequate induction programme can facilitate movement between the role of lecturer and practice educator. A practice educator wishing to teach primarily in higher education would be required to examine the lecturer programme outcomes and determine areas for professional development. In the same way a lecturer wishing to move into a practice-based teaching role would follow an induction programme specifically tailored to meet developmental needs arising from such a change in focus.

Continued professional development

Activity 4.13

What is continued professional development and in what way could your own attitude towards continued professional development affect the learning experience of students placed with you?

Continued professional development is a concept that has become well established in the nursing profession in recent years. It refers to the recognition of need for ongoing opportunities for learning and development beyond the point of initial qualification. The Institute of Personnel and Development stated that the point of registration should represent 'an endorsement of an individual's fitness for practice', with the proviso that professional updating is an ongoing process.[25] Continued professional development is signified by recognition that the achievement of a professional qualification in nursing is the entry point to a new phase of learning, rather than the end of the process. It encourages practitioners to continue to think about their practice and continually seek better ways of working. The benefits of continued professional development impact on the individual practitioner and the quality of the learning experience subsequently offered to students. It has a major contribution to make in relation to high standards of practice in terms of:[25]

- keeping up to date with changing circumstances and requirements
- maintaining an openness to new ideas and new perspectives
- adopting an approach based on critical reflectivity
- maintaining an open mind in order to guard against prejudice and discrimination
- providing an ongoing source of stimulation and motivation
- a series of opportunities for mutual support and shared learning
- a basis for team work and team development
- a safeguard against burnout.

Thompson *et al.* suggest that without a commitment to continued professional development there is a danger that staff will practise in a routine, uncritical way, losing sight of the values and knowledge base that underpin practice.[26] Practitioners in this situation should not be mentors. As the role of mentor is pivotal to the learning experience of the student, it is crucial that they establish a commitment to continued professional development. The requirement to keep abreast of new developments is exemplified by the UKCC who state, 'As a registered nurse, midwife or health visitor, you are personally accountable for your practice and in the exercise of your professional accountability, must ... maintain and improve your professional knowledge and competence.'[27] The statutory requirements for the implementation of the UKCC's post-registration education and practice (PREP) came into force on 1 April 1995. This means that since April 1998 all registered nurses, midwives and health visitors have to demonstrate that they have met the PREP requirements when they renew their registration. Alongside a number of other requirements the UKCC specifies that in order to maintain registration each individual nurse, midwife or health visitor must:

- complete five days of study activity
- maintain a personal professional profile.

To meet the needs of patients and students there is an obligation on the part of practitioners not only to maintain and extend existing capabilities but also to acquire new knowledge and skills to respond to the rapidly changing healthcare environment in which they work.

Conclusion

Within this chapter a range of issues related to assessing students in clinical practice have been explored. Whilst the discussion relates to the mentor's role in supporting and assessing students in practice, the issues discussed can be used by practitioners to assess the effectiveness of their mentoring.

Activity 4.14

Reflect for a moment on what you have read in this chapter.
How can you use what you have read in this chapter to improve your own performance as a mentor?

Seeking comments and feedback from students will help you evaluate your role and performance as a mentor. Additional feedback on your performance as a mentor can be sought by eliciting the views of your peer group (colleagues and other mentors). The latter can be undertaken informally or in a more structured way using peer review or assessment. Sharing experiences with colleagues in this way can help you to identify additional knowledge and skills that you may require, leading to a plan of action which gives direction to your continued professional development activities. The section on portfolios may have set you thinking about your responsibilities regarding the development of your own professional portfolio. After all, it is difficult to espouse the virtues of portfolios if you haven't yet started your own.

> ## Activity 4.15
>
> Review your own professional development portfolio and learning needs.
> Update it in the light of the work you have undertaken within this chapter.

In a climate where the workload is continually increasing with deadlines to meet and targets to achieve, the time available to assess students may diminish. The UKCC was critical of the organisation and supervision of students on placements within pre-registration programmes, suggesting that this was compounded by pressure of work and the pace of activity in healthcare environments.[1] It is important to remember that in the final analysis, the assessment you undertake not only determines the diplomas, degrees and future careers of students, but it also determines the quality of future healthcare delivery in this country.

References

1 UKCC (1999) *Fitness for Practice*. UKCC, London.

2 UKCC (2000) *Requirements for Pre-Registration Nursing Programmes*. UKCC, London.

3 Rowntree D (1987) *Assessing Students: how shall we know them?* Kogan Page, London.

4 Quinn FM (1997) *The Principles and Practice of Nurse Education*. Stanley Thornes, Cheltenham, p. 229.

5 English National Board (1986) *Devolved Final Written Examinations*. (1986/30/ERDB). ENB, London.

6 Redman W (1994) *Portfolios for Development: a guide for trainers and managers*. Kogan Page, London.

7   Brown RA (1992) *Portfolio Development and Profiling for Nurses.* Quay Publishing, Lancaster.

8   English National Board (1997) *Standards for the Approval of Higher Education Institutions and Programmes.* ENB, London.

9   Liverpool John Moores University (2000) *School of Health and Human Sciences DIP HE (Nursing) Clinical Briefing Pack.* LJMU, Liverpool.

10 Jarvis P and Gibson S (eds) (1989) *The Teacher Practitioner in Nursing, Midwifery and Health Visiting.* Chapman and Hall, London, p. 83.

11 Philip T (1983) *Making performance appraisal work.* McGraw-Hill, Maidenhead.

12 Couchman W and Dawson J (1990) *Nursing and Health Care Research: a practical guide.* Scutari Press, London, p. 52.

13 ENB and DoH (2001) *Placements in Focus: guidance for education in practice for health care professions.* ENB and DoH, London.

14 Gallego A and Walter P (1991) Preparation of health care teachers for the future. *Nurse Education Today.* **11**: 94–9.

15 Charnock A (1993) The personal tutor: a teacher's view. *Nursing Standard.* **7**: 28–31.

16 Jowett S, Payne S and Walton I (1994) *Project 2000. The Final Report.* NFER, Slough.

17 Liverpool John Moores University (2000) *School of Health and Human Sciences DIP HE (Nursing) Validation Document.* Vol. 1, June 2000, p. 62.

18 ENB and DoH (2001) *Preparation of Mentors and Teachers: a new framework of guidance.* ENB and DoH, London.

19 Camiah S (1998) Current educational reforms in nursing in the United Kingdom and their impact on the role of nursing lecturers in practice: a case study approach. *Nurse Education Today.* **18**: 368–79.

20 Philips R (1994) Providing student support systems in Project 2000 nurse education programmes: the personal tutor role of nurse teachers. *Nurse Education Today.* **14**: 216–22.

21 Bewley C (1995) Clinical teaching in midwifery – an exploration of meanings. *Nurse Education Today.* **15**: 129–35.

22 Gibbon C and Kendrick K (1996) Practical conflicts. *Nursing Times.* **92**: 51–5.

23 ENB and DoH (2001) *Preparation of Mentors and Teachers: a new framework of guidance.* ENB and DoH, London.

24 UKCC (2000) *Standards for the Preparation of Teachers of Nursing, Midwifery and Health Visiting.* UKCC, London.

25 Institute of Personnel and Development (1996) *Continuing Professional Development: a guide to 'doing' CPD*. North Cheshire and North Wales Branch, IPD Merseyside, p. 34.

26 Thompson N, Murphy M and Stradling S (1994) *Dealing with Stress*. Macmillan, London.

27 UKCC (1992) *Code of Professional Conduct*. UKCC, London.

CHAPTER FIVE

Getting it right: the legal and professional aspects of assessment

Bridgit Dimond

Chapter overview

- Introduction
- Accountability – civil, employer, professional, criminal
- Human rights
- Appeals processes
- Contractual rights of the student
- Health and safety issues
- Responsibility of the mentor for the student
- Beverley Allitt situation
- Issues of character confirmation
- Record keeping
- Whistle blowing
- Conclusion

Introduction

State registration is the most important protection for the general public against incompetent, dishonest and dangerous healthcare practitioners. The legal entrance onto the register kept by the UKCC is therefore extremely important in ensuring that only those on whose competence and integrity the public can rely are entitled to be placed on the register. (Note that in April 2002 the Nurses and Midwives Council (NMC) will be established and will provide a new framework for statutory registration of nurses, midwives and health visitors. In addition it will take on a new role in relationship to healthcare assistants.) In this chapter the legal aspects relating to the role of the mentor as one who helps determine a student's clinical competence are considered. However, it must also be remembered that often the mentor's role combines a number of functions. Frequently the mentor takes on teaching, supervision, and instructing responsibilities and each of these have their own specific legal repercussions. It is clearly essential that mentors obtain an unambiguous description of their responsibilities, so that there can be no dispute over what specific tasks they should be undertaking.

Accountability – civil, employer, professional, criminal

Accountability is a continuous process of monitoring professional performance which should aim to be at the highest level of skill and competence. Accountability therefore is to patients or clients, the public at large, the employer, the governing body and to oneself. Healthcare professionals are answerable for their own action or omission, they cannot consider that someone in higher authority will assure accountability for their error because they were acting on behalf of someone else.

Consider the following exercise: what do you think are the implications for the mentor in the following scenario?

Activity 5.1

A mentor is not satisfied that a student has reached a satisfactory standard by the end of the placement. Nevertheless, a satisfactory grading is given on the student's summative assessment.

A mentor could face several different forums of accountability as a result of grossly negligent conduct. These will be considered briefly, but reference should be made to more detailed works setting out the legal points.[1]

Civil liability: Bolam Test standards of assessment

The most obvious concern for the mentor is the possibility of being challenged on the grounds that the assessment was unfair. What standard would be required of the mentor? How could he or she defend him or herself?

The courts would apply the Bolam Test if there were any dispute over what standards should have been used in any assessment. This derives from a case in 1957[2] where the judge ruled that in assessing professional negligence the following principle should be followed:

> 'The standard of care expected is the standard of the ordinary skilled man exercising and professing to have that special skill.'

This means that in a dispute over assessment standards, expert evidence would be given over what would be seen as reasonable practice by a competent mentor assessing a student in those specific circumstances. Mentors must be able to justify their marks; giving an unduly low mark would be as negligent and professionally unacceptable as giving a higher mark than justified.

The duty of care in the law of negligence also includes the duty to take care in giving information. For example mentors sometimes state that they would not fail a student on clinical placement because they 'do not want the hassle of having to explain to an appeals panel why they have done so'. In this situation passing an unsatisfactory student is failing to take care in the giving of information and is therefore a negligent act.

There can be liability if information is given negligently, in the knowledge that it will be relied upon by a recipient, if as a result of that reliance the recipient suffers harm. This is further discussed under the section on references (*see* p. 112). However, consider the following example which illustrates this point.

Activity 5.2

A mentor signs a student's clinical skills record to say that he or she is proficient in taking blood pressures. On the student's next allocation his or her new mentor reads the clinical skills record and delegates the task of taking blood pressures to the student. Unfortunately the student is not competent in this skill and fails to perform the task correctly, resulting in inaccurate observations.

This may have repercussions, not only on the student and the patient, but also for the second mentor whose reputation for responsible delegation may be called into question.

Employer and contract of employment

Another way in which mentors are accountable relates to their contract of employment. Most mentors are employees and therefore would be expected to obey the reasonable instructions of the employer and to act with reasonable care and skill. These requirements are implied terms in the contract of employment. A dispute over what is a reasonable instruction may sometimes arise, and it would clearly be unacceptable for an employer to require a mentor to act unfairly or to act in any way which was contrary to reasonable standards of practice. If a mentor failed to obey reasonable instructions, i.e. to assess a student's performance, or act with reasonable care and skill in doing so, he or she could be disciplined with the ultimate sanction of dismissal. This could be challenged at an employment tribunal if the employee considered that the dismissal was unfair.

Professional accountability

Consider the following exercise: what do you think are the implications for the mentor in the following scenario?

Activity 5.3

Sometimes students complain that their mentor has a personal dislike of them, and believe that an unsatisfactory assessment may result for this reason.
If the complaint is substantiated what might be the implications for the mentor?

Mentors must be objective in their assessment of students. This issue is discussed more fully in Chapter 4 (*see* p. 84). Personal animosity or personality conflicts which are allowed to influence assessments invalidate the results of the assessment. In addition, if it is shown that a particular mentor has acted out of malice or has shown personal animosity to a student, then he or she could face disciplinary action or professional conduct proceedings, and also his/her employer could be held vicariously liable for the actions of the assessor. A mentor who is registered with the UKCC (or after April 2002 the NMC) would face professional conduct proceedings if she or he had failed to abide by the Code of Professional Conduct with the ultimate sanction of removal from the register. Any evidence that the mentor favoured one student unduly or victimised a student, or was in breach of confidentiality (see below) could be followed by professional conduct proceedings.

Criminal liability

Criminal proceedings are unlikely as a consequence of the work of a mentor, but in exceptional situations fraudulent practices by an assessor could result in criminal proceedings. For example, a mentor may be offered a bribe to enable a student to pass her exams and to be entered onto the register. Such conduct would be aiding and abetting a criminal offence and therefore could be followed by prosecution in the criminal courts.

Mentors may be involved in criminal cases even though they are not personally charged with an offence. For example in a case such as that of Beverley Allitt, where a former student is subject to criminal proceedings, the evidence of the mentor might be required in relation to the conduct and history of the student.

Human rights

Since 2 October 2000 the European Convention on Human Rights has been directly enforceable in the courts of England and Wales (and in Scotland from the date of devolution). All public bodies must ensure that they comply with the Articles set out in the Convention and mentors are responsible for ensuring compliance in their own work. The following text highlights Articles of significance to the role of the mentor.

Article 3 of the European Convention on Human Rights states that:

> 'No one shall be subjected to torture or to inhuman or degrading treat-
> ment or punishment.'

It is hoped that mentors would actively encourage a positive relationship
with those subject to their assessment and that they would treat them
with dignity and humanity. It would be an extreme situation where a
mentor could be challenged for a breach of Article 3. However it could
arise that the student brings to the mentor's attention concerns relating
to inhuman or degrading treatment that he or she had witnessed at work
and the student sought the mentor's advice in deciding what action should
be taken. This is a potential whistle blowing situation (*see* p. 113).

Article 5 of the European Convention on Human Rights states that:

> 'Everyone has the right to liberty and security of person. No-one shall
> be deprived of his liberty save in the following cases and in accordance
> with a procedure prescribed by law.'

This is an article which may give rise to concerns if the mentor becomes
aware that patients who are not detained under the Mental Health Act
1983 are being kept inappropriately in locked rooms. Detention in such
circumstances may be justified at common law (i.e. judge-made law),[3]
but the circumstances of temporarily locking someone up who is not
detained under the Mental Health Act 1983 should be regularly reviewed.
This is another Article which could lead to a whistle blowing situation.

Article 6 of the European Convention on Human Rights states that:

> 'Individuals have the right to a fair trial.'

This right will have significant implications since it applies not just to
criminal charges but also to the determination of civil rights and obligations. It would therefore apply to disciplinary actions and other such
forums, where at present employees may not have representation and
they may be in a very weak situation compared with the employer. The
mentor as an employee is entitled to have a fair hearing if involved in disciplinary proceedings with the employer. The rights of the student are
considered under appeals. Article 6 is relevant.

Article 8 of the European Convention on Human Rights states that:

1   'Everyone has the right to respect for private and family life, his home and his correspondence.'
2   'There shall be no interference by a public authority with the exercise of the right except such as is in accordance with the law and is necessary in a democratic society in the interests of national security, public safety or the economic well-being of the country, for the prevention of disorder or crime, for the protection of health or morals, or for the protection of the rights and freedoms of others.'

Activity 5.4

A mentor does not have a very high opinion of a student, and expresses it to mentors from other clinical areas to which the student might be allocated in the future. Is the mentor in breach of any law or professional code of conduct?

It would therefore be a violation of Article 8 if a mentor discussed a student and the assessment of the student in circumstances where there was no professional justification for that disclosure. The decision to share or withhold confidential information, however, may be influenced by a variety of factors. Consider, for example, the mentor's responsibilities in the following scenario.

Activity 5.5

A student informs the mentor that she has had to seek psychiatric advice because of an ongoing problem, but was not intending to discuss this with the staff at the university because she did not want anyone to know of her illness.

In taking appropriate action the mentor needs to take into account the Code of Professional Conduct which states that as a registered nurse . . . in the exercise of your professional accountability, you must:

'report to an appropriate person or authority, having regard to the physical, psychological and social effects on patients and clients, any circumstances in the environment of care which could jeopardise standards of practice.'[4]

In this scenario the mentor might consider the student to be potentially liable to jeopardise standards of practice and might consider that this information should be made available to his or her own manager. Ideally the student would be directed to discuss the problem with the appropriate university staff. This may be the student's personal tutor, the student welfare department or the occupational health department. In the latter case it may be left to the occupational health doctor to decide on what action should be taken. This situation gives rise to considerable concerns since the case of Beverley Allitt (see p. 110).

Article 14 of the European Convention on Human Rights states that:

'The enjoyment of rights and freedoms set forth in this Convention shall be secured without discrimination on any grounds such as sex, race, colour, language, religion, political or other opinion, national or social origin, association with a national minority, property, birth or other status.'

Whilst Article 14 does not give a right in itself, it protects all those who are claiming rights under any of the other articles from discrimination. The examples given of forms of discrimination, whilst extensive, are not exhaustive, and other forms of discrimination such as those based on age could be added to the list. This Article should also be read in conjunction with the Disability Discrimination Act 1995. Any student or member of staff may have a claim if they suffer discrimination by the organisation or colleagues and other individuals. Both the educational institution and the organisations offering clinical placements should ensure that policies against discrimination are in place and implemented.

Action possible under the Human Rights Act 1998

Any student who considers that his or her rights have been infringed by a mentor could sue the employer of the mentor in the civil courts, seeking judicial review of the decisions and actions of the mentor. In addition the rights of the Convention also apply to the mentor, who may be able to allege a violation of Article 14 by the employer.

Appeals processes

Each education or training institution must ensure that there is a robust, equitable, accessible and just system of appeals. Article 6 is of particular importance in the assessment process, since it is fundamental to any appeals process where results of the assessment or the actual carrying out of an assessment is challenged. Mentors should ensure that if there is a challenge to their assessment, they ensure that an independent person reviews the situation and the appropriate appeals machinery is enacted. The principles of natural justice would require that any person involved in hearing an appeal is independent and impartial, hears the evidence from the appellant and ensures that the decision made is in accordance with the evidence received. The decision of an appeals hearing could be challenged in the High Court by way of judicial review if there is an allegation that the principles of natural justice have not been followed or if there is an alleged breach of Article 6. The Appeals process should also cover the timing of assessments and examinations. For example, if a mentor fails to carry out an assessment in time to give the student an opportunity for rectifying any shortcomings (and such an opportunity should have been made available to the student), then the student may well have grounds for appeal. This is discussed further in Chapter 4 (*see* p. 84).

Activity 5.6

One of the difficulties often faced by mentors is that their shifts do not always coincide with those of their students; sickness or holidays may also interfere with the assessment process. How can the mentor ensure that the student is fairly assessed under these circumstances? What legal or professional principles apply?

Clearly a mentor cannot be on duty at all times when the person subject to the assessment is working. It is of concern to mentors that, because of the extent of their duties, they are simply taking a snapshot of the competence and abilities of the person being assessed. There may be circumstances which arise when the mentor is not present which would suggest that the student may not be suitable for inclusion on the register or for passing a particular module. In order to plan for these circumstances it is important that the mentor establishes a safe system of assessment, so that actions taken when the mentor is not present are reported to the mentor. This may mean that some of the assessment may be delegated to others provided that they have the necessary education, training and competence.

Contractual rights of the student

Because the student is not qualified and therefore not on the professional register, their act or omission has to be investigated by their Trust, the training institution and the professional body which validate their training programme. Students have to be held responsible in law for their actions in the same way as members of the public are responsible. Although a higher level of accountability lies with the registered practitioner, students must be aware of their responsibility to carry out nursing care in a safe and skilled manner.

The student may have in law a contract of services with the higher education institution (HEI). Where fees are paid by or on behalf of the student, then rights under a contract of services may arise. For example if the student claims that he or she has received very poor supervision or teaching, then there may be contractual rights which are enforceable against the HEI authority as well as rights enforceable in the law of negligence if harm has occurred.

Health and safety issues

A mentor would be subject to the duties under the Health and Safety Act 1974, particularly section 7, and the employee's duty to take reasonable care of his own health and safety and that of others and also to assist the employer in complying with health and safety regulations. The mentor may also be involved in assessing practice and techniques used in health and safety situations such as manual handling. The records of the mentor may be relevant to any case brought in respect of a back injury at work.

Responsibility of the mentor for the student

> ### Activity 5.7
>
> To what extent are you, as a mentor, responsible for a student's actions?

There is no concept of vicarious liability for a senior person for the actions of a junior unless the former is an employer of the latter. However, negligence may arise if the mentor has negligently delegated activities to the student which are outside the student's competence, or has failed to ensure that the appropriate level of supervision is given to the student. Reasonable precautions should be taken to ensure that the student works within their sphere of competence at times when the mentor is not personally present.

Beverly Allitt situation

Beverly Allitt, an enrolled nurse, was convicted of murdering four children, of attempting to murder three others and of causing grievous bodily harm to six more. She was sentenced to life imprisonment on every count. An independent inquiry chaired by Sir Cecil Clothier made significant and substantial recommendations on the selection procedures for nurses, including the prohibition of employment of those with a personality disorder.[5] The Clothier Report recommended that there should be a review of sickness information being referred to occupational health and for the criteria for the management of referrals to occupational health; there should be untoward incident reports if there is a failure of an alarm on monitoring equipment; and reports of serious untoward incidents should be made in writing to district and regional health authorities. The Department of Health drew the attention of NHS managers to the report's recommendations.[6] The report accepted that no measures can afford complete protection against a determined miscreant and stated that:

> 'Our principal recommendation is that the Grantham disaster should serve to heighten awareness in all those caring for children of the possibility of malevolent intervention as a cause of unexplained clinical events.'

Clearly each mentor must bear in mind the possibility that a student may suffer from a personality disorder and ensure that the recommendations contained in the Clothier Report are implemented.

Issues of character confirmation

Success in practical and theoretical assessments are not the only requirement for entry on to the UKCC register.[7] The UKCC also requires confirmation of good character for inclusion on the register. A form is issued which has to be completed by the head of the school (or department) of nursing within the HEI, making a declaration that there is no reason why the student is not eligible to be placed on the UKCC register. This places a clear duty on the mentors to ensure that any information which indicates that the student would be unsuitable should be brought to the attention of the head of the school or department of nursing. This requirement is particularly important in the light of the recommendations of the Clothier inquiry into Beverly Allitt (see above).

If a student is told that he or she cannot continue the course, this may be justified on the grounds that the head of the school or department of nursing would not be able to sign a good character form at the end of the course. Conversely, a school may become liable to the student if it fails to remove a student from the course and, after three years of training and after the student has passed the practical and theoretical modules, refuses to sign the character form. The school may be challenged by the student because he or she was kept on the course, even though the head of the school or department of nursing knew that he or she would not get registration. In such circumstances the student may have a right of legal action. Had the school made known its view on the suitability of the character of the student, then the student would have left the course and not wasted his or her time in finishing the course only to be refused registration.

Record keeping

It should be clear from what has been said that there are many occasions when the records of the mentor might be required in evidence. Minimum information should be kept to ensure that questions can be answered about any assessment and the students involved. Such information would include:

- the names of those being assessed, with details of location, grade, etc.
- the times and dates of the assessment
- the content of the assessment
- the grades of achievement and any comments by the assessor
- action taken by the mentor.

Placement reports and statements

Activity 5.8

What status do a mentor's written comments have in law?

Liability can arise when a mentor writes a report. If a report is written negligently then liability can arise both to the recipient of the report, if in reliance upon that report she or he has suffered harm[8] and also to the person who is the subject of the report.

Providing a reference

Activity 5.9

A mentor is asked to provide a reference for a student who has had a warning at work for losing his temper. The student asks the mentor not to refer to this incident assuring her that he now has his temper under control. What is the position if the mentor gives the reference without mentioning this incident, and the student obtains a post and then the employer blames the mentor for an inaccurate reference which has led to harm?

If the character of the student was relevant to the use the recipient would make of the reference, then it should have been mentioned in a reference, and if it is omitted, then the mentor could be liable for negligent advice. In such circumstances, she should either have told the student that she could not give a reference without mentioning the incident or she should have told the student that if she gave a reference it would have to include a mention of the incident.

On the other hand, there can also be liability to the person on whose behalf the reference is given, if the reference is written without reasonable care and if harm occurs to the subject of the reference as a result of potential employers relying upon the reference.[9] Every care should be taken to ensure that it is written accurately in the light of the facts available. If a reference is given with due care and is defamatory of the individual, the writer of the reference should be protected from any successful action of defamation, regardless of whether the comments are correct or incorrect, provided they were given in a qualified privileged situation without malice by the writer.

Whistle blowing

Activity 5.10

A student witnesses what she or he perceives to be unacceptable practice and reports it to a higher authority. As a member of staff who has participated in, or condoned, the practice, how does the law require you to behave towards the student?

A student may witness unacceptable practice whilst on a placement, or the student might report to the school that he or she has major concerns about practice or health and safety matters. The Public Interest Disclosure Act 1998 provides protection for the whistle blower against any victimisation resulting from such concerns being raised and the Department of Health requires all health organisations to introduce a procedure to implement the Public Interest Disclosure Act 1998.[10]

Conclusion

This chapter has aimed at setting out the basic principles of law which apply to the role of the mentor. Clearly not every possible legal concern which could arise has been discussed, but the mentor is referred to the sources of information given under further reading. It should be remembered too that law is a dynamic area and mentors should keep up to date as new statutes are enacted and cases heard.

References

1 Dimond B *The Legal Aspects of Nursing* (3e). Pearson Education, (in press).

2 *Bolam v. Friern Hospital Management Committee* (1957) 1 WLR 582.

3 *R. v. Bournewood Community and Mental Health NHS Trust ex p L* (1998) 3 All ER 289; (1999) AC 458.

4 UKCC (1992) *Code of Professional Conduct*. UKCC, London.

5 Clothier Report (1994) *The Allitt Inquiry*. An independent inquiry relating to deaths and injuries on the children's ward at Grantham and Kesteven General Hospital during the period February to April 1991. HMSO, London.

6 DGM (1995) 71 *The Allitt Inquiry*.

7 UKCC (2000) *Requirements for Pre-Registration Nursing Programmes*. Registrar's letter, 17 May.

8 *Hedley Byrne v. Heller and Partners Ltd*, House of Lords. (1963) 2 All ER 575.

9 *Spring v. Guardian Assurance PLC and others*. *Times Law Report*, 8 July 1994.

10 Department of Health HSC 1999/198 *Public Interest Disclosure Act 1998*.

Further reading

Kennedy I and Grubb A (2000) *Medical Law and Ethics* (3e). Butterworth, London.

McHale J, Fox M and Murphy J (1997) *Health Care Law*. Sweet and Maxwell, London.

McHale J, Tingle J and Peysner J (1998) *Law and Nursing*. Butterworth-Heinemann, Oxford.

Montgomery J (1997) *Health Care Law*. Oxford University Press, Oxford.

Skegg PDG (1998) Law, *Ethics and Medicine* (2e). Oxford University Press, Oxford.

Tingle J and Cribb A (eds) (1995) *Nursing Law and Ethics*. Blackwell Science, Oxford.

Tschudin V and Marks-Maran D (1993) *Ethics: a primer for nurses*. Bailliere Tindall, London.

Vincent Charles *et al.* (1993) *Medical Accidents*. Oxford University Press, Oxford.

Vincent Charles (ed) (1995) *Clinical Risk Management*. BMJ Publishing, London.

Wilkinson R and Caulfield H (2000) *The Human Rights Act: a practical guide for nurses*. Whurr Publishers, London.

Young P (1989) *Legal Problems in Nursing Practice*. Harper and Row, London.

Young, AP (1994) *Law and Professional Conduct in Nursing* (2e). Scutari Press, London.

CHAPTER SIX

An effective placement: creating a learning environment

Bob Swann

Chapter overview

- Introduction
- Components of an effective learning environment
- Motivating factors for students and staff
- Applying Maslow's hierarchy of needs – a framework for analysing the learning environment
- Auditing the learning environment
- Conclusion

Introduction

Initially we considered entitling this chapter 'A popular placement – creating an effective learning environment'. However, after reflecting on our personal experiences and through discussions with experienced practitioners and current students we reached the point of questioning whether 'popular' was necessarily synonymous with 'effective'. We remember placements within our own nursing programmes which were popular with students, but it is unlikely much effective learning took place. Whilst it is important, wherever possible, for learning to be enjoyable, it is evident that students have in the past learned and will in the future learn from situations which may not seem enjoyable.

The importance of the quality of practice placements in the education of healthcare professionals is emphasised in *Making a Difference* and is an integral part of the Department of Health's drive to modernise the NHS.[1] Within this, considerable attention is paid to strengthening education within healthcare, focusing on the needs of patients and clients. As practice placements account for 50% of the curriculum within pre-registration programmes, it is essential that they are able to provide a supportive environment where effective learning can take place.

Defining the clinical learning environment is not straightforward. Quinn described it as a holistic notion involving every aspect of a clinical setting involving the student themselves.[2] This broad definition takes into account a range of factors that may influence the quality and the effectiveness of the learning environment. Managers, mentors, preceptors, clients and patients all have a part to play in influencing the environment. Other influences include the systems in the workplace and the student's capacity to integrate and work within them. In practice, it is either difficult or artificial to separate these aspects. However, for the purposes of exploration and learning, this chapter separates and considers some of the key components. Having explored these, we suggest a framework which provides ways of thinking about, organising and subsequently working towards audit of those factors essential to an effective learning environment.

Components of an effective learning environment

Our first consideration of the learning environment stems from a number of nursing research studies which identify students' perceptions of the main characteristics of an effective learning environment.[3-5] The studies make reference to the importance of an atmosphere that recognises the needs of the employee. Whilst students are not direct employees of the placement provider, the impact of working with a staff group who do not feel valued and supported by their employers cannot be overstated. Orton concluded in her research that the quality and management strategies of the ward sister were influential in creating a highly student-oriented ward.[3] These studies collectively identified that team spirit, a humanistic approach to students, management style, teaching and learning support were key factors in the creation of an effective learning climate. Whilst much of this research relates to hospital environments, the principles can be readily applied to all care areas. Before reading any further consider the following exercises.

Activity 6.1

What do you understand by the terms 'team spirit' and 'humanistic management styles'?

Team spirit, humanistic approach and management style

Team spirit is an elusive concept, although it is logical to assume that team spirit can only be developed from genuinely working as a team. Sisson suggests the term 'team working' has come to be used in a variety of ways and contexts.[6] Many would see team working arising from a work situation where the interests of the employee and the organisation are seen to be one and the same, leading to the necessity rather than just the requirement that everyone works as a team. Another view of team working refers to a *team at work* where people from a variety of backgrounds in terms of training, education and primary role, come together to produce a particular service. This aspect of team working is particularly evident within current approaches to healthcare which emphasise multidisciplinary working, supported by the pooling of budgets and shared education and training.

Team working is best achieved where managers encourage a sense of group pride and self-esteem across all levels and disciplines. Staff should receive just rewards for their contributions with managers showing a genuine concern for staff welfare. In effect, managers should create a feeling of mutual trust and respect with staff. A team approach, with an appropriate leadership style on the part of the manager, creates fertile ground for the development of an appropriate learning climate.

Climate can be described as the prevailing atmosphere surrounding the organisation where learning takes place. It includes the level of morale and strength of feelings or belonging and goodwill among members. Tagiuri and Litwin defined organisational climate as 'a relatively enduring quality of the internal environment of an organisation that is experienced by its members, influences their behaviour, and can be described in terms of the values of a particular set of characteristics (or attributes) of the organisation'.[7] The place in which you work is characterised by the relationships between senior and junior staff and their relationship with the organisation as a whole. These relationships, in turn, are determined by the interactions between formal structure, processes of management, styles of leadership and the behaviour of the people working within the organisation.

Whilst each organisation has distinctive features Mullins suggests that a healthy organisational climate might exhibit the following characteristics:[8]

- the integration of organisational goals and personal goals
- the most appropriate organisation structure based on the demands of the socio-technical system
- democratic functioning of the organisation with full opportunities for participation
- justice in treatment with equitable personnel and employee relations policies and practices
- mutual trust, consideration and support among different levels of the organisation
- the open discussion of conflict with an attempt to avoid confrontation
- managerial behaviour and styles of leadership appropriate to the particular work situations
- the acceptance of a psychological contract between the individual and the organisation
- recognition of people's needs and expectations at work, and the individual differences and attributes
- equitable systems of rewards based on positive recognition
- concern for the quality of working life and job design
- opportunities for personal career development and career progression
- a sense of identity with, and loyalty to, the organisation and a feeling of being a valued and important member.

Activity 6.2

How may these organisational climate factors affect the quality of the learning environment?

A healthy organisational climate is likely to provide an effective learning climate. Knowles identified a learning climate as one in which 'adults feel at ease [physically] ... psychologically being accepted, respected and supported ... the existence of a spirit of mutuality between teachers and the students as joint enquirers ... in which there is freedom of expression without the fear of punishment or ridicule ... known by name, and valued as a unique individual'.[9]

At either extreme the organisational climate can either encourage an atmosphere where staff and students can learn or discourage any opportunity for growth and development. A humanistic approach acknowledges people as individuals as well as team members. Faugier supports this humanistic approach in her proposition of a *growth and support model* which contains elements related to generosity of time and spirit, openness, willingness to learn, sensitivity and trust.[10] If staff feel their efforts are not valued or relationships within the organisation are poor, this in turn will have a profound effect on the quality of the learning experience for both staff and students. All staff within the organisation have a responsibility to work together effectively as a team, ideally encouraging students to feel part of that team.

Teaching and learning support

Teaching and learning support mechanisms within the placement will have a significant impact on the amount and quality of learning that takes place. An effective placement should provide students with a structured learning experience including an opportunity to receive comprehensive orientation to their placement, an induction programme and opportunities to learn from a wide experience. Students should be supported by staff who are willing to take on the role of mentor, supervisor and assessor. Such staff should have an appropriate attitude, experience, qualifications and preparation for teaching, assessing, support and supervision roles. In addition they should also be able to demonstrate commitment to their own continued professional development.

Facilitating learning is of the utmost importance and clinical staff need to be familiar and skilled in the use of a variety of strategies. Self-directing strategies such as problem-based learning (PBL), for example, provide the student with the opportunity for guided discovery learning.

Whilst there are a number of recognised approaches to implementing PBL, it is frequently used within the university setting to assist students to bridge the gap between theory and practice. As a strategy, PBL seeks to give students control over their own learning in the context in which it will be used. It encourages open-minded, reflective, critical and active learning[11] and seeks to develop highly competent practitioners who will continue to learn effectively throughout life.[12] Familiarity with PBL as a learning strategy will help staff to facilitate the students' learning more effectively. Other self-directed learning strategies focus on encouraging students to determine individual learning needs through self-assessment and portfolio development. These latter strategies are discussed in more detail in Chapter 4. All of these learning strategies are designed to encourage the student to take an active rather than a passive role in their learning and are aimed at stimulating reflection, analysis and critical thinking. Students should be encouraged to take an active responsibility for their own learning. The atmosphere should encourage the development of critical thinking and provide a culture where students can observe staff challenging each others' practice in a supportive environment and where they themselves can question practice without feeling guilty or disloyal.

The availability of learning resources, such as access to the Internet, literature from relevant journals, books and access to patients' notes also helps the student to increase their understanding of patients' needs. A designated area of study is also advantageous and allows the student to concentrate on specific tasks which may be more readily undertaken in quiet surroundings.

Whilst the quality of nursing care is not synonymous with the quality of the learning environment, a placement delivering poor quality care would be of dubious value to student nurses. Students should experience the positive culture of clinical governance, where practice is founded on relevant research and evidence-based findings. Provision of care is underpinned by sound theoretical knowledge which informs practice and is, in turn, informed by practice.

Activity 6.3

What human and material resources in your clinical area are available to help students learn?
Are these resources readily available and accessible to students?

Motivating factors for students and staff

One of the essential requirements for learning to take place is motivation. Within the care area we are seeking to provide not only a positive environment but also the motivation to learn. Whilst the student is the focus of this chapter, it should be acknowledged that a dynamic learning environment can only be created and perpetuated by staff who are equally willing to learn. Motivating people is a complex issue and has been the subject of a proliferation of techniques, all of which have sought to improve employee motivation. Techniques such as facilitated supervision, quality circles, total quality management (TQM), performance awards and performance-related pay are just a few examples. Buchanan and Huczynski define motivation as 'the internal psychological process of initiating, energising, directing and maintaining goal-directed behaviour'.[13] They suggest motivation can be self-initiated and also influenced by the actions of others, through such things as encouragement, praise or even intimidation. Motivation is about satisfying people's needs and wants; once they feel it is worthwhile doing something, satisfaction is generated and they are ultimately motivated to repeat positive experiences.

Biological and physical make-up also creates forces that influence much of our behaviour. These physiological needs or forces are known as 'drives' and are activated by deprivation. Drives are recognised as relentless activity that leads to behaviour designed to reduce needs. For example, if we are hungry we need food, if we are thirsty we need a drink. Motives on the other hand are learned needs. Discussions in Chapter 4 confirm that values, ideals and beliefs shape our motives and ultimately our behaviour, leading us to pursue particular goals because they are socially valued. A great deal of what we do, in terms of how we think and behave, is shaped by the society to which we belong. In essence, motives are learned, have a social basis, are activated by environment and aimed at stimulation. Drives, however, are innate, have a physiological basis, are activated by deprivation and aimed at satiation. Within this explanation we have drawn an artificial line between biological drives and socially acquired motives. In the 'real world' there is considerable overlap between the two. By way of example we may need to drink; however, we may want an expensive wine. We may need the wine to quench our thirst and want the wine for the pleasure of its taste, for its intoxication, or for what it says about us in terms of social status. These thoughts and decisions will not always be at a conscious level and we will not always be clear in our minds as to what extent we are satisfying wants, needs and drives.

There does, however, appear to hierarchy or order to these drives and motives. Maslow suggested that ans have eight innate needs (*see* Box 6.1).[14–16]

Box 6.1 Maslow's Hierarchy of Needs

Transcendence needs: spiritual.
Self-actualisation needs: development and realisation of capabilities and potential to their fullest.
Aesthetic needs: for order and beauty.
Knowing and understanding needs: curiosity, learning, philosophising, experimenting, exploring, the need to gain and systematise knowledge.
Esteem needs: confidence, achievement, self-respect and self-esteem, independence, reputation, prestige.
Affiliation needs (often referred to as social needs): attachment, sense of belonging, affection, love, friendship.
Safety needs: safety and security, freedom from pain or threat of physical attack, protection from danger, shelter and order.
Biological needs: homeostasis (the body's automatic efforts to retain normal functioning), oxygen, food, water, sunlight, rest, sleep, sexual desire.

Maslow suggests that some of these needs will have lower priority until other specific needs have been satisfied.[15] The biological and safety needs are at the base of the hierarchy and satisfaction of these needs is vital to survival. When these needs are effectively met, individuals will move in search of higher order needs and for some this will lead ultimately to self-actualisation and transcendence. Maslow also maintained that a need is not an effective motivator until those needs lower in the hierarchy are satisfied. When people are hungry, thirsty, cold, or afraid, for example, they are less likely to be concerned about higher order needs. If you are starving or being chased by a rabid dog, you will not be interested in the aesthetics of your surroundings. Maslow went on to explain that a satisfied need is no longer a motivator. The needs of the next level in the hierarchy become the motivating influence and demand satisfaction. In other words, if you have just eaten you are unlikely to be motivated by food.

Self-actualisation and transcendence can be seen as the high points of human fulfilment. You will note that in Table 6.1, transcendence – the fulfilment of spiritual needs – has been omitted as it is beyond the remit of this text, self-actualisation being enough of a challenge. Self-actualisation is seen as a postulated need for growth, continual self-development and the realising of potentialities. Maslow claims self-actualisers have 'peak experiences' which they seek to repeat.

Activity 6.4

Which factors provide the greatest motivation for you in your work: recognition, status, relationships, responsibility, financial reward, working conditions?

What do you think are the key motivating factors for some of the students who are placed with you?

Table 6.1 A framework for analysing the learning environment

Hierarchy of needs	Factors within the clinical learning environment	Insert your own ideas
Self-actualisation	• Positive challenges • Achievable tasks and assignments • Opportunity to use initiative and creativity • Opportunity to reach synthesis	
Aesthetics	• Well-designed working environment in terms of buildings, structure, décor, gardens, natural light, etc. • Environment that is encouraging and rewards creativity	
Knowing and understanding	• Opportunities to learn using different methods • Access to evidence-based practice • Reflective practice and learning • Access to information • Open communication • Constructive feedback • Clinical supervision	

Table 6.1   (*continued*)

Hierarchy of needs	Factors within the clinical learning environment	Insert your own ideas
Esteem	<ul><li>Recognition</li><li>Confidence</li><li>Status</li><li>Praise and reward</li><li>Positive feedback from colleagues, superiors, mentors and preceptors</li></ul>	
Affiliation	<ul><li>Feel valued and part of a cohesive team</li><li>Friendly supervision</li><li>Positive communication</li><li>Networking, relationships</li><li>Individuals feel they have a contribution to make</li></ul>	
Safety and security	<ul><li>Safe working conditions</li><li>Policies and procedures</li><li>Compliance with health and safety legislation</li><li>Control Of Substances Hazardous to Health (COSHH)</li><li>Controls assurance standards</li><li>Clinical Negligence Scheme for Trusts (CNST)</li><li>Adequate repairs to building</li><li>Appropriate staffing level and skill mix</li><li>Ensuring theory and practice are integrated</li><li>Student-centred teaching and learning</li><li>Orientation programme for new staff and students</li><li>Identified mentors and preceptors</li><li>Peer support</li><li>Development of trusting relationships</li></ul>	
Biological requirements	<ul><li>Adequate salary to provide for an adequate diet, living accommodation, etc.</li><li>Pleasant working conditions</li><li>Adequate tea and meal breaks</li><li>Canteen facilities with affordable meals</li></ul>	

Applying Maslow's hierarchy of needs – a framework for analysing the learning environment

Maslow's hierarchy provides a useful framework for considering how the clinical learning environment might satisfy each level of need for staff members and students alike. The list identified in Table 6.1 is by no means exhaustive and is intended as a starter to which you can add your own ideas.

People are motivated by a variety of needs and wants. For some the satisfaction that there are better outcomes which equate to the amount of effort they put into the job will be the motivating factor. Others will be motivated by status or money. Motivation is about sustaining commitment, support and enthusiasm. Recognition and appreciation of work performance is crucial. It is important to highlight good practice and not just focus on things that go wrong since the latter, if handled inappropriately, can foster a blame culture. We need to take a positive approach to adverse healthcare events, learning lessons from incidents and from near misses.[17]

Auditing the learning environment

Having considered the factors that contribute to creating an effective learning environment, a comprehensive picture begins to emerge. *Knowing* these things in itself is not enough, we have a responsibility as mentors and placement providers to ensure they *exist* with a degree of consistency in the areas for which we have responsibility. We are fortunate in that many if not most of these influences can be identified, observed and subsequently measured. The vehicle for achieving this is audit. This section provides the building blocks, enabling you to contribute towards the development of a learning environment audit tool, tailored to your own practice area. Haigh *et al.* suggest that the process of audit is a way of 'gaining a snapshot or statement of affairs'.[18] In educational terms audit is an effective way of reviewing current activities and learning opportunities available to students during practice placements.

Introducing the concept of audit in relation to learning environments may not, in the first instance, be greeted with universal approval. Evans noted 'many still see the use of performance indicators as a most threatening activity. We must encourage our staff to develop positive attitudes for whatever their views, this approach is here to stay.'[19] Although written some 14 years ago, this statement holds true today, perhaps even more so given that audit has become an established part of all NHS organisations and is a central component within the delivery of evidenced-based practice.

Hallet and Thompson suggest that there are a number of key stages to getting audit right and these include:[26]

- getting the culture right in the first place
- having measurement systems in place that everyone owns and understands that reflect true success, and are properly managed and driven
- having an educational forum for discussing developments and setting standards
- having a regular reporting mechanism.

Shailer goes on to suggest that prior to the development of any audit tool, it is essential that careful consideration is given to:[21]

- available research in the use of performance indicators
- evaluation of previous audit related to the learning environment
- research conducted in the area of learning environments
- discussions with clinicians, lecturers and practice educators in order to clarify values and philosophies, relating these to the objectives of the organisation.

As within any area of practice which seeks to evaluate the effectiveness of a particular system, in the first instance, it is useful to determine whether the information gained from existing audit tools is as accurate and relevant as it needs to be. Existing audit systems may be outdated and unfit for the purpose. There is a proliferation of literature regarding audit and the learning environment and a tool developed by another organisation can frequently be adapted to suit local circumstances. In addition to this, you will no doubt be influenced by the exercises you have undertaken whilst reading this chapter.

Activity 6.5

Obtain a copy of the last educational audit report for your own clinical area.

What does this snapshot tell you about the learning environment at that particular time?
Since the time of the last audit what things have changed to affect the quality of student learning?

At this point it is important to acknowledge the underlying principles involved in providing appropriate practice placements. The English National Board (ENB) and Department of Health (DoH) identifies the need for robust partnership between service providers and practice educators working together with students. Each member of the partnership must ensure that placements offer the expected opportunities for learning and that each student's practice experience contributes to the learning outcomes consistent with the aims of the education programme. They identify four checklists aimed at those organisations responsible for practice placements. The checklists focus on:

- providing practice placements
- the practice learning environment
- student support
- assessment of practice.

Whilst not exhaustive, these checklists provide a useful basis for both informal and formal assessment or audit exercises within the organisation. You may wish to refer to the guidance document for more detailed help. However, Box 6.2 contains an abridged version of the combined lists which may be useful to practitioners wishing to reflect on the suitability of the learning environment within their own practice area.

Box 6.2   Placement area checklist

- Does the area have a stated philosophy of care which is reflected in practice and supports curriculum aims?
- Does the practice provision reflect respect for the rights of health service users and their carers?
- Does the provision of care reflect respect for the privacy, dignity and religious and cultural beliefs and practices of patients and clients?

- Is care provision based on relevant research-based and evidence-based findings where applicable?
- Does care provision involve different models of care commensurate with current practice and encompassing local and national initiatives?
- Are interpersonal and practice skills fostered through a range of teaching/learning methods?
- Does the practice experience enable students to experience the role of the registered practitioner in a range of contexts?
- Do all placements have an infrastructure to support continuing professional development opportunities for practitioners?
- Do students gain experience as part of a multiprofessional team?
- Is a resources area available in the practice environment?
- Does student feedback contribute to the ongoing evaluation of the learning environment and the student experience and are all stakeholders aware of the feedback?
- Do placement providers have a profile which determines:
  - maximum number of students at any time in the placement
  - the skills required by the student before beginning the practice experience
  - the learning opportunities available and the learning outcomes expected from the placement?
- Have practitioners working in the practice area received preparation for their role in teaching, supporting and supervising students?
- Do mentors know what the student is expected to achieve through specified practice outcomes?
- Does the practice placement enable students to experience the full 24 hours a day, seven days per week nature of healthcare delivery?
- Is the practice placement audited in line with the requirements of the statutory/professional body as to their continuing suitability for students' practice experience?
- Is good practice disseminated following audit and monitoring and does joint action planning address areas of concern and areas needing enhancement?
- Are students given an initial interview during the first week of the placement, to agree the learning outcomes and ways of achieving them, taking into account their prior knowledge and experience?

- Are students' learning needs, achievements and opportunities reviewed regularly?
- Does the experience available among clinical staff support the students' achievement of the learning outcomes of the educational programme at the appropriate level?
- Do students receive consistent supervision and support during the practice placement?
- Is there a named assessor with qualifications and experience commensurate with the context of care delivery and the requirements of the appropriate professional and statutory bodies who supervises and guides students in the practice placements?
- Do practice staff have dedicated time in educational activities to ensure they are competent in teaching and mentoring roles?
- Are students assisted with linking theory to practice?
- Is the student's practice assessed within the context of a multi-professional team?

Activity 6.6

Think about your workplace as a learning environment. What would be the first thing you would do to bring about improvements? Draw up a list of achievable steps aimed at prioritising and implementing your improvements.

The audit process is ongoing. Once the initial audit is undertaken, the information obtained is analysed and disseminated. Any changes need to be agreed within the team and subsequently implemented. It is essential that re-audit takes place after a given time to determine the effects of these changes. Student participation in the auditing process is useful and can be achieved in a number of ways. The student can be requested to complete a questionnaire at the end of their placement. The questionnaire may be geared towards the overall effectiveness and quality of the delivery of care and it can be aimed at the students' perception of the quality and effectiveness of the learning environment. There is also a role for students in relation to the development of an appropriate audit tool and this may be achieved through membership of an appropriate subgroup of the overall curriculum-planning team.

Conclusion

The essence of this chapter is to encourage you to consider the learning environment and to understand the fundamental impact you can make on the overall opportunities for students to learn. As the old saying goes 'you can take a horse to water, but you can't make it drink'. To an extent this applies to students in the workplace, they must come to the placement with the desire to learn. It can be seen, however, that with some forethought and a structured approach we can create the most 'fertile ground' for learning to take place. Within this chapter we have explored the preparatory work necessary in the practice placement area and developed an understanding of the audit process.

Creating a learning environment can be likened to undertaking a journey. Before embarking on any journey it is a good idea to know where you want to go. Of even greater importance is that you need to know where you are starting from. The baseline audit helps us to realise where we are starting from. Where we are going is influenced by our service objectives and underpinning philosophy. The audit process will enable you to chart your progress in the development of a learning climate. As well as looking forward, it is also important to look back and recognise all the things we have achieved. The audit gives you the capacity to do this. We can often take for granted the tremendous progress made within the area of delivery of care and support for students, and looking back can be a boost to morale and confidence for staff and student alike.

At the beginning of the chapter, we reflected on placements within our own programmes of preparation for nursing. It is important for you to do the same. In preparing any learning environment, it is essential to consider the student and their perspectives. After qualifying it is all too easy for us to lose sight of how it feels to be a student, the sometimes overwhelming amount of information to take in and the pressure to perform, both in the university and in the service area.

As a final note, it is important for us to recognise that we are all learning together and that learning is a continuous process. The delivery of care is a dynamic ever-changing process requiring staff and students to continue learning throughout their careers. Not only is learning together the most effective approach it can also be the most enjoyable. In essence the creation of an effective learning environment is of benefit to everyone – students, staff and most importantly those people receiving our care and support.

References

1   DoH (1999) *Making a Difference: strengthening the nursing, midwifery and health visiting contribution to health and health care*. DoH, London.

2   Quinn F M (1988) *The Principles and Practice of Nurse Education* (2e). Chapman and Hall, London.

3   Orton H (1981) *Ward Learning Climate*. Royal College of Nursing, London.

4   Fretwell J (1982) *Ward Teaching and Learning: sister and the learning environment*. Royal College of Nursing, London.

5   Ogier M (1982) *An Ideal Sister: a study of the leadership style and verbal interactions of ward sisters with nurse learners in general hospitals*. Royal College of Nursing, London.

6   Sisson K (1995) *Personnel Management: a comprehensive guide to theory and practice in Britain*. Blackwell Business, Oxford, p. 641.

7   Tagiuri R and Litwin GH (eds) (1968) *Organisational Climate*. Graduate School of Business Administration, Harvard University, p. 27.

8   Mullins LJ *Management and Organisational Behaviour* (4e). Pitman Publishing, London, p. 717.

9   Knowles MS (1970) *Androgogy: an emerging technology for adult learning*. In: M Tight (ed) Adult Learning in Education. Croom Helm, London, in association with the Open University, pp. 53–70.

10 Faugier J (1992) In: T Butterworth and J Faugier (eds) *Clinical Supervision and Mentorship in Nursing*. Chapman and Hall, London.

11 Glen S and Wilkie K (2000) *Problem-Based Learning in Nursing: new model for a new context?* Macmillan Press, London, Chapter 2.

12 Boud D and Feletti GI (eds) (1997) *The Challenge of Problem Based Learning* (2e). Kogan Page, London.

13 Buchanan D and Huczynski A (1997) *Organisational Behaviour: an introduction text* (3e). Prentice Hall, London, pp. 68–72.

14 Maslow AH (1943) A theory of human motivation. *Psychological Review*. **50**: 370–96.

15 Maslow AH (1954) *Motivation and Personality*, Harper and Row, New York.

16 Maslow AH (1994) *The Farther Reaches of Human Nature*. Penguin Books, Harmondsworth.

17 DoH (2000) *An Organisation with a Memory: report of an expert group on learning from adverse events in the NHS*. HMSO, London.

18 Haigh D (1995) A person-centred approach to education audit. *British Journal of Nursing.* 4: 838–41.

19 Evans L (1987) Performance Indicators in Nurse Education. *Senior Nurse.* 7: 7–9.

20 Hallet L and Thompson M (2001) *Clinical Governance: a practical guide for managers.* Emap Public Sector Management, London, p. 90–91.

21 Shailer B (1990) Clinical Learning Environment Audit. *Nurse Education Today.* 10: 220–7.

CHAPTER SEVEN

Learning from experience: enabling students to benefit from reflection

Chapter overview

- Comparison of humanist and behaviourist approaches to learning
- The nature of reflective practice
- Kolb's experiential learning cycle as a clinical learning tool
- A reflective account example
- Students' preferred learning styles
- Capitalising on students' strengths and developing their weaknesses through experiential learning

The humanistic approach to learning advocated by such people as Rogers and Knowles sees the student as a person with the potential for self-directed learning who will learn whatever is meaningful to him or herself.[1,2] Clearly, in any form of professional education, students require the guidance of experts and cannot be left entirely to their own devices in terms of determining their own learning outcomes. The question, in the context of nurse education, is one of balance. To what extent should learning be controlled and how may the students' natural inclination for self-directed learning be utilised for self-development?

A feature of professional education and practice in recent years has been the prominence given to the notion of reflective practice. Nurses, midwives and health visitors are among groups such as social workers and teachers who have embraced reflection as a means of enhancing professional practice. The purpose of this chapter is to clarify the concept of reflective practice, discuss the conditions necessary for its effective use, explore its potential in clinical nurse education, and consider how you, as a mentor, can help your students to benefit from the technique.

In contrast to the behaviourist approach discussed in Chapter 2, the process of reflection cannot be controlled so easily, nor can its outcomes be easily prescribed. One of the central tenets of the humanistic philosophy is that individuals are unique and interpret their environment in a unique way. That is to say they will decide what is meaningful and important within whatever context they happen to be in at the time. The challenge to mentors is to ensure that suitable learning experiences are available at appropriate times and are sufficiently interesting to motivate the student to actively engage with them; active engagement necessarily involves reflecting on personal experience.

Despite its apparent popularity, doubt exists about the degree of understanding of the concept amongst the professionals who claim to use it. In her paper provocatively entitled *The Reflective Practitioner: mantra or model for emancipation*, Ecclestone suggested that the term reflection is often used without sufficient understanding of its complexity, perhaps being chanted repetitively without thought being given to its real meaning.[3]

Experiential learning

In his description of experiential learning, Kolb refers to the cyclic process in which a 'concrete experience', i.e. an actual event in someone's life, is followed by reflective observation (Figure 7.1).[4]

Reflection is a systematic analysis of an experience, although in our experience of teaching nurses on pre- and post-registration courses, it is sometimes a poorly understood concept. It is often perceived as a remembrance of an event and the feelings it generated, rather than an analysis. We often look back on life events and think 'that was good, I enjoyed it', or 'I didn't like what happened ... I felt really uncomfortable about it'. These are remembrances, not reflections. Fitzgerald says that learning through reflection is 'laborious and deliberate ... not something done in the head on the way home. It is an analytical process which may be uncomfortable and lead to personal distress and conflict.'[5]

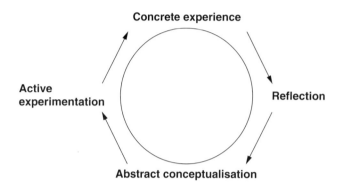

Figure 7.1 Kolb's experiential learning cycle.

An analysis is a structured process, so in order to reflect, rather than just remember, a structure is necessary. A number of structures, or models, of reflection have been prepared and it is a matter of personal choice as to which one is selected. Boud *et al.* developed a three-phase model based on the process of reflecting on *actions*, *feelings* and *knowledge* which we have adapted and includes a *skill* component, as nursing students obviously need to develop skills as well as knowledge.[6] The student considers the actions involved in the event and what the various players, including themselves, did. At first the consideration is descriptive but it can lead to thoughts such as 'Why did I do this' or 'What would have happened if she had done that?' Then there is consideration of the feelings generated by the experience. Boud *et al.* state that unless negative emotions are dealt with, further learning is inhibited.[6] Conversely, positive emotions may lead to a desire to seek out similar experiences leading to the competence that comes with practice and the development of new insights.

The third component of this reflective model is knowledge and skills. The individual reflects on the relevant knowledge and/or skills they used in an event, which reinforces its value and retention. However, significant personal development occurs when the individual recognises what they do *not* know about the event, or what they *cannot* do.

Following the reflection stage, according to Kolb's model, is a process of consolidation and confirmation of new knowledge and insights (abstract conceptualisation), to which we would add the refining of skills. At this stage new knowledge and skills are added to the student's repertoire.

The next stage, active experimentation, is when these are tried out in the next similar situation the student engages in. If successful the student may be described as competent at the skill, but at this stage not yet expert. Expertise is acquired by repeatedly going through the cycle until performance is consistently good and the underpinning knowledge has been internalised.

Activity 7.1

The following section is an extract from the reflective diary of Keith, a nursing student who wrote about his experiences while on his first clinical placement.

Try to identify what learning he has achieved in each of the following areas: knowledge, skills and attitudes.

An extract from the reflective diary of a nursing student

The area of physiological measurement I am going to reflect on . . . is the taking and measuring of blood pressure. These measurements were taken on my first placement, which is a ward of 18 elderly mentally ill patients who are suffering from functional illnesses rather than organic. . . . The patient I was taking the blood pressure from had a long history of hypertension and postural hypotension so it was important that the nursing team had regular readings until the medication took effect. I carried out a series of blood pressure readings over a period of four days. The blood pressure readings were done with the patient sitting and standing to enable the staff to see if there was any postural drop in blood pressure. These are the results that followed:

	Sitting (mmHg)	Standing (mmHg)
Day 1	160/120	160/100
Day 2	170/120	165/100
Day 3	170/110	155/90
Day 4	165/110	155/90

These results indicated that this person was suffering from hypertension and postural hypotension . . .

The results below were recorded after the patient had been taking the prescribed medication for 14 days. These readings were over a specific number of days and showed that the medication was starting to work.

	Sitting	Standing
Day 1	190/90	190/80
Day 2	145/85	130/80
Day 3	170/80	170/80
Day 4	165/80	150/80

Deficits

The first knowledge deficit I noticed I had when I was placed on the ward was that I was not aware of the difference between a functional illness and an organic illness.

When attempting to take blood pressure from a patient I found that I felt a little awkward when approaching the patient, I felt that I was invading his privacy in some way especially when having to take hold of him personally and move his arm. However, I now find that with the practice I have been receiving I am able to complete the task without feeling I am intruding on the individual.

When I first tried to take the patient's blood pressure I found it nearly impossible to locate the systolic/diastolic readings. The main problem that I had was not being able to locate the stethoscope over the brachial artery in the crease of the arm. I had to try this on several different patients before I found it for the first time and then I began to become more confident with the more patients that I tried.

Other deficits I recognised while looking after this patient were that I had very little experience in looking after people who were suffering ongoing physical ailments as well as mental problems. I also recognised that it was much harder to communicate with people who are suffering from depression and anxiety because a symptom of these illnesses can be social withdrawal and apathy, which can make it difficult for the staff to get to know the patient and strike up a rapport. I also found that I knew relatively nothing about blood pressure readings and the importance of keeping them stable and what the meaning of diastolic and systolic pressure meant.

Knowledge

Systolic is the reading that you gain when the heart is expanded and there is maximum pressure on the artery. Diastolic is the pressure on the artery when the heart is at rest (O'Brien and O'Malley 1982). By gaining the reading of both systolic and diastolic, usually on three different occasions, we can assess whether the patient needs further investigations. If the patient does require medication to regulate their blood pressure they will be prescribed antihypertensive drugs. These are split in to four groups:

Diuretics which decrease fluid and salt in the circulation.
Beta-Adrenoceptor blocking drugs which slow the heart.
Vasodilators which widen the blood vessels.
Drugs that work on the nervous system (O'Brien and O'Malley 1982).

After reading some literature and gaining some practical experience I found that I was able to hear the Korotkoff sounds when taking blood pressure. These sounds are named after the Russian surgeon Korotkoff who classified these audible sounds into five phases. My understandings of this method are as follows:

1   Tapping that is sharp and clear.
2   Blowing or swishing.
3   Sharp but softer than phase one.
4   Muffled and fading.
5   No sound.

This individual patient was on a number of different medications but one was primarily for the control of his blood pressure. The medication that the patient took to regulate blood pressure was Ramipril. Having seen the patient prescribed the medication and take it, the blood pressure readings did drop down to a more acceptable level. The medication that was prescribed is named ACE, which stands for angiotensin converting enzyme, inhibitors, which act on the heart and the blood vessels. They inhibit the conversion of angiotensin 1 to angiotensin 2, and are effective and well tolerated (BNF 1999).

The skills I had when I started to care for the patient were that I had a lot of experience in communicating with patients who were suffering from mental illnesses and I was also very good at reassuring them and I could listen to a person's history and problems without becoming judgemental.

Action plan

The plan of action I took to address my skill and knowledge deficits was as follows. When there was an opportunity to take blood pressure readings I would ask to become involved so that I was gaining more experience in handling and approaching patients. This then gave me more experience in trying to locate the brachial artery, which I did find difficult at first.

There were numerous books that I consulted to enhance my awareness about the differences between an organic illness and a functional illness. I also approached several different professional staff over the course of my placement to see if they could give me any other information.

The way I addressed the problem of having no experience in looking after people who had physical, as well as mental, problems was to become involved in dialogue with the patients.

To gain more knowledge and information in understanding the meaning of systolic and diastolic blood pressure and how the various medications worked I attended the library on several occasions and perused through the relevant books on this subject. I also consulted the Drug Information Unit at my placement and they gave me some interesting information.

New skills

My understanding now of the importance of monitoring a person's blood pressure is that there could be serious complications if this is untreated. Guidotti and Jobson (1992) clearly state that:

'Blood pressure is often wrongly measured and recorded in both developed and developing countries.' (Guidotti and Jobson 1992: 1)

As a result of this there could be a CVA (cerebral vascular accident) or a stroke. This is where an artery in the brain bleeds causing paralysis and other problems. Smith (1991) states:

'Pressure can also cause heart disease and hardening of the arteries. This happens because the arteries have to change to cope with the additional pressure; the inner linings become rough, the walls thicken and the diameter of the artery narrows. The blood flow then becomes sluggish so it clots easier so then may be causing a thrombosis (Smith 1991: 22)

Medical professionals are concerned that people who are hypertensive run the risk of increased early mortality (Sadik and Elliot 1999).

Through talking to different professionals and some literature searching I have now found out that blood pressure is constantly changing and is influenced by emotional and environmental factors. These factors make it difficult to obtain an accurate measurement of blood pressure, which is why blood pressure is measured over a specific period to enable us to gain a more precise reading (O'Brien and O'Malley 1982). Williams (1997) also cites:

'There is evidence that hypertension is very common in patients with diabetes.' (Williams, 1997: 20)

Having undertaken this reflection I have found that people who are elderly and suffering from physical ailments as well as mental illness require a lot of support and encouragement to go about their daily routine.

Having never taken blood pressure before I now feel confident in this task and I am able to use the equipment effectively and interpret some of the results.

Another new skill that I have acquired has been the way that I communicate with and approach patients. I have a gained a gentler approach when dealing with patients, especially the elderly. I now take my time to explain the procedure that I am undertaking and make sure that they feel comfortable and not threatened by my actions.

I am also now aware of the difference between a functional illness and an organic illness. A functional illness is when a patient complains of symptoms for which no physical cause can be found. An organic illness is associated with changes in the structure of an organ (McFerran 1998).

(For reference details *see* p. 148.)

You will see from this account that the simple everyday activity of measuring a blood pressure offers the student a wide range of learning opportunities. The word constraint on his assignment did not allow Keith the opportunity to discuss issues such as the physiology of the cardiovascular system, or the legal aspects of record keeping.

Interestingly it also shows how conventional academic structures may limit a student's development. As a first-year student Keith's learning should have been at Level 1, the acquisition of knowledge and development of understanding concepts. The analysis that he demonstrated in interpreting a series of blood pressure recordings is an activity normally associated with Level 2. Rosenthal and Jacobson once wrote about the 'self-fulfilling prophecy' in education;[7] if we believe that students can only learn up to a certain level, and restrict our teaching to within that level the students will not learn beyond it, thus 'proving' that they did not have the ability to progress beyond it in the first place. By allowing students to engage in meaningful learning, i.e. what is significant to them at the time, the barriers are removed and learning is under the students' control.

Activity 7.2

Read through his account again and map out his progress against Kolb's experiential learning cycle.

Using Kolb's cycle as a model we can see that Keith's *concrete experience* was the measurement of the blood pressure of a vulnerable elderly mentally ill patient. His *reflection* focused on three areas:

- the action of taking the blood pressure
- his sensitivity and feeling of invading the patient's personal space
- his lack of knowledge of certain physical and mental illnesses, and the realisation that he already had the relevant skills for communicating with elderly mentally ill patients that he had acquired through previous work.

For Keith two important things emerged from this experience. First, it allowed him to acknowledge what knowledge and skill he already had. This is an important motivational factor; it creates a 'feel-good' effect and even a sense of self-worth as a team member (compare this with Maslow's self-esteem stage in Chapter 2). This encourages students to move on to the next sphere of learning (compare this with Vygotsky's scaffolding notion, also in Chapter 2). Second, it enabled him to diagnose his own learning needs. You will see from his action plan that he set about addressing what he described as his 'knowledge and skill deficits'. He took ownership for his own learning needs and the responsibility for doing something about it. These actions, stemming from his reflections, contribute to his new knowledge and insights, or in Kolb's terms, an *abstract conceptualisation*. Additionally, he developed his skill in measuring blood pressure.

Reflective preferences of nursing students

We said earlier that reflection is sometimes a poorly understood concept. This is despite the fact that research by one of the authors has shown that nurses, both qualified and unqualified, have a fairly strong predisposition to reflect (*see* Figure 7.2) according to a survey using the Honey and Mumford Learning Styles Inventory.[8]

Although this representative sample shows that most nursing students have this high predisposition for reflection, it does not necessarily follow that they will reflect on practice. Because someone can do something it does not mean that they will do it. (We all have the potential to perform criminal acts but relatively few of us do.) In order for potentials to develop, the right conditions must exist to nurture them. Discussions with those who participated in the study indicated that they neither had the time during working hours, nor the support of a mentor. A study undertaken

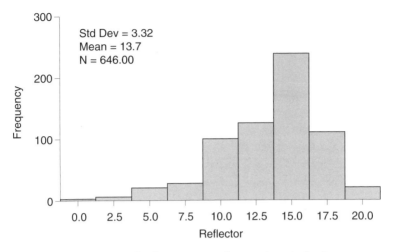

Figure 7.2 The distribution of reflector scores for nursing students.

by Welsh *et al.* showed that, despite being taught a framework of reflection, most nurses were not able to describe it when asked how they encouraged students to reflect on practice.[9] This strengthens the view that the necessary conditions for effective reflection do not always exist in clinical practice.

Another condition, as seen in Keith's reflective account, is the use of a reflective model; this gave structure to the reflection and allows for the descriptive element to proceed through analysis to synthesis, the development of new insights or skills. However, this could not happen unless there was an investment in time; to reiterate Fitzgerald, who said that learning through reflection is 'laborious and deliberate ... not something done in the head on the way home'.[5] It is clear from Keith's account that a considerable amount of time was spent in deliberating over the aspects of his experience. He also said that he approached several different professional staff over the course of his placement to see if they could give him any other information. In other words, the support of people with expertise is valuable; as a mentor you are in a position to direct your student to relevant sources (people, literature) if you do not have sufficient knowledge yourself. Or you can act as the moderator, the person who assesses whether or not the student's understanding is accurate, and corrects him or her if it is not.

So far then, we have seen that the use of students' own experiences can generate learning. Kolb said that 'learning is the process whereby knowledge is created through the transformation of experience'.[4] Kolb was referring to *personal* knowledge as opposed to *propositional* knowledge. Propositional knowledge is secondhand – passed on from teachers, books, etc. Through reflecting on experience the student does not just know *about* something, their knowledge is at a deeper level. The four conditions for effective reflection are as follows.

1   The individual's predisposition to reflect.
2   The use of a structured framework for reflection.
3   Sufficient time to give to the process.
4   The support of a mentor.

Activity 7.3

With reference to the UKCC outcomes and competencies (*see* Appendix), how can you create situations for your students which will help them to meet the requirements for a competent practitioner in your own clinical area?

Developing other facets of professional practice

The Honey and Mumford Learning Styles Inventory is an instrument which assesses four dimensions of a person's character.[8] We have already referred to the reflective dimension, but it is worth considering the activist, theorist and pragmatist dimensions.

Activists prefer to be involved with practical activities, and learn through doing.
Theorists prefer intellectual activities such as reading and discussing ideas.
Pragmatists prefer to roll their sleeves up, get on with a task and see what happens. They have little time for reflective activity, in contrast to the **reflector** discussed earlier who takes a more cautious approach and likes to think things through before commitment to anything.

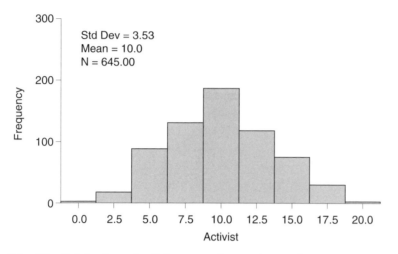

Figure 7.3   The distribution of activist scores for nursing students.

Figures 7.3, 7.4 and 7.5 show the distribution of scores for nursing students of these three remaining facets of professional practice. In each case the mean scores show only a moderate predisposition for these learning styles. This is a concern for two reasons. First, nursing is a practical activity and we would hope that students would have a stronger inclination to this aspect of their course. Second, it is desirable that, as university students, they should have more than a moderate inclination towards theoretical activities.

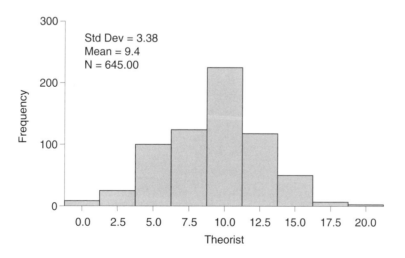

Figure 7.4   The distribution of theorist scores for nursing students.

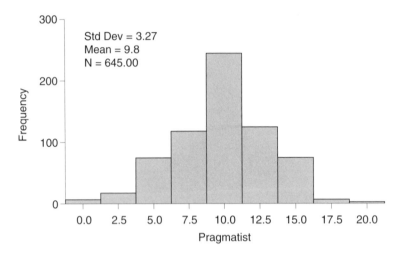

Figure 7.5   The distribution of pragmatist scores for nursing students.

Summary

In this chapter we have attempted to show how you, as a clinical nurse, can capitalise on the students' innate ability to learn, and their motivation to do so, by utilising the wide range of clinical experience which is available in your area. Learning can still take place even when you are under severe workload pressure. Although teaching can be a labour intensive activity, the role of mentor does not mean that you necessarily have to give direct tuition all the time. It is worth looking at a concept described by Race (*see* Figure 7.6), which refers to high and low teacher inputs and high and low student gains.[10]

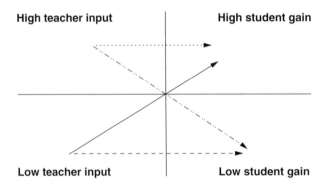

Figure 7.6   Teacher inputs and student gains.

It is possible to put a lot of effort into teaching students; however, they may still not learn as much as hoped. Conversely little effort (not no effort) may result in a high level of learning. The amount of learning Keith demonstrated resulted from relatively little teacher input. At the beginning of the chapter we said that students require the guidance of experts. Your role is to help students to select appropriate learning experiences, ensuring that guidance and support are available (not necessarily from yourself) and to provide the time and expertise to aid their reflection. In doing this you are contributing to the conditions for effective learning, i.e.:

- drawing on the students' predisposition to reflect
- facilitating the use of a reflective model
- providing the time for the students to reflect
- acting as a mentor to share your knowledge and expertise, correct any misconceptions or faulty techniques the student may have, and assess their levels of learning.

This process will also address the other concerns identified in the research into students' preferred learning styles. Figures 7.3 to 7.5 show only a moderate predisposition for learning through doing (activist) or for engaging in intellectual activity (theorist). You will be encouraging the students to participate meaningfully and to develop their intellect through exploration of the theoretical principles which underpin their practice. This linking of theory and practice is likely to encourage the students to be more confident in their approach to nursing (pragamatism).

Above all, by encouraging the student to reflect on practice you will be helping them to close the theory–practice gap and contribute to their development as 'knowledgeable doers'.

References

1   Rogers CR (1983) *Freedom to Learn for the 80s*. Merrill, New York.

2   Knowles M (1990) *The Adult Learner: a neglected species*. Gulf Publishing, New York.

3   Ecclestone K (1995) *The Reflective Practitioner: mantra or model for emancipation*. Prescription or Reflection? Liberating the Competence Model in Post-Compulsory Education Conference, University of Central Lancashire, 26 October.

4   Kolb D (1984) *Experiential Learning: experience as the source of learning and development.* Prentice Hall, New York.

5   Fitzgerald M (1994) *Theories of Reflection for Learning.* In: AM Palmer, S Burns and C Bulman. *Reflective Practice in Nursing.* Blackwell Scientific, Oxford.

6   Boud D, Walker D and Keogh R (1985) *Reflection: turning experience into learning.* Kogan Page, London.

7   Rosenthal R and Jacobsen L (1968) *Pygmalion in the Classroom: teacher expectation and pupils' intellectual development.* Holf, New York.

8   Honey P and Mumford A (1992) *The Manual of Learning Styles.* Peter Honey, Maidstone.

9   Welsh I, Napier NR, Richardson G *et al.* (1998) Is the ENB Course 998 Fit for Purpose? *Nurse Education Tomorrow.* Ninth International Conference, University of Durham.

10 Race P (2001) Developing Assessment Strategies Workshop. Liverpool John Moores University, Liverpool.

Extract references

- *British National Formulary* (1999) BMA and RPSGB, London.

- Guidotti R and Jobson D (1992) *Detecting Pre-Eclampsia: a practical guide.* WHO, Geneva.

- Hogston R and Simpson PM (eds) (1999) *Foundations of Nursing Practice.* Macmillan, London.

- McFerren AT (1998) *Oxford Mini Dictionary for Nurses* (4e). Oxford University Press, Oxford.

- O'Brien E and O'Malley K (1982) *High Blood Pressure and What it Means to You.* Dunitz, London.

- Smith T (1991) *Living with High Blood Pressure.* Sheldon Press, London.

- Williams B (1997) *Diabetes and Hypertension: a fatal attraction explained.* Initiative Books, Kent.

CHAPTER EIGHT

Working in partnership

Chapter overview

- Introduction
- Staff exchanges between education and service providers
- Joint appointments
- Research activities
- Conclusion

Introduction

Throughout the history of the NHS, some 53 years, the pace of change has varied. It is fair to say, however, that the present pace of change is far greater than at any other period over this time. There is no single reason for this, rather a number of factors that have come into play. Rapid technological change, particularly within the field of computing and word processing, makes the whole process of change that much easier and faster. It is unlikely, given these technological advances, that the pace of change will ease. It is more likely that the situation will exist where rapid change is ever present and becomes the normal state of affai. Alongside these technological advances, changes have taken place with regard to the delivery of care and the provision of education.

Healthcare needs are invariably complex and their effective del beyond the capacity and competence of any single profession, a discipline. Managing change effectively and efficiently dep collective endeavour in which partnerships play a crucial r that effective partnerships between higher education insti and practice are both desirable and essential. For these be successful there must be joint planning and delivery of services with a parallel collaboration between service and education in the planning and delivery of educational programmes. These partnerships are central to the objectives embedded within key documents such as *The New NHS: modern, dependable*,[1] National Service Frameworks for Mental Health,[2] Coronary Heart Disease,[3] and Older People,[4] the *NHS Plan*[5] and *Valuing People: a strategy for learning disability*.[6] It is also clear that for partnerships to be successful, budgets must be pooled and services combined, and the way forward for this was created within the 1999 Health Act. Clearly, working in partnership, whilst being appropriate and desirable is also a political imperative.

Education and health providers have a long history of working together and in many instances mechanisms for collaborative working are already well established. Opportunities to involve all providers within the health and social care economy should continue to be developed, as working together in this way facilitates the sharing of expertise, ideas and perspectives. The end product is also then a needs-driven education *and* service-led curriculum reflecting the complexity of current service delivery.

Acknowledging the wider context for working in partnership along with the associated issues and key driving forces, it is necessary to explore the tasks and relationships integral to working in partnership. Joint curriculum development, for example, is likely to encourage common ownership of programmes, increasing the likelihood of success through joint investment. Mentors responsible for students in the practice setting are more likely to be familiar with assessment strategies if they have been ᵕlved in the developmental stages. In the same way, the presence of ᵕtaff on the curriculum team is more likely to facilitate the devel- ᵕᵕement outcomes that can be realistically achieved in the ᵕʰis understanding of each other's view of the 'health- ᵕt the student's experience in the classroom is ᵕ takes place in the practice environment, ᵕ together.

ᵕᵕum also involves the determina- ᵕce staff involved in curriculum ᵕscuss the advantages and disad- ᵕgies, some of which are relatively ᵕl learning (PBL) strive to encourage ᵕ problem solving, analysis and synth- ᵕrs who have an understanding of the ᵕch they live and practice. In essence it helps to develop practitioners who can handle ambiguity and change. Familiarity with these new approaches is fostered through the involvement of practice staff in the curriculum-planning process, in turn, leading to the effective implementation of new learning strategies in practice.

A common theme highlighted within this book is the joint responsibility of practitioners and educators to create and offer high quality teaching and learning opportunities for students and to monitor their effectiveness. The quality and degree of support offered to students influences their ability to gain effective practical skills and ultimately provide the care needed by patients and clients. Chapters 4 and 6 explore these issues at length and provide valuable guidance for ensuring both education- and practice-based staff are able to provide structured learning opportunities for students along with the required level and quality of support.

Staff exchanges between education and service providers

As previously discussed, education and service providers working together on particular projects enhances understanding of each other's roles and responsibilities. A logical extension to working on joint projects is the provision for staff exchanges between the respective institutions. Staff exchanges should be viewed as developmental and an exciting opportunity for learning. However, the aim should be to provide this type of developmental opportunity without disrupting the current level of performance within the exchanging organisations.

The requirement to maintain credibility in both education and practice was highlighted by Burnard and Chapman[7] and more recently by the UKCC.[8] Recommendation 26 of *Fitness for Practice* states that 'service providers and HEIs should support dedicated time in education for practice staff and dedicated time in practice for lecturers, to ensure that practice staff are competent in teaching and mentoring roles and lecturers are confident in the practice environment'.[8] 'Job swops' of this nature, however, can be difficult to organise. In the current climate of rapid change and complex objectives, it is difficult to spare 'experts' to be replaced by someone with relatively less skill and understanding.

However, we must seek to manage these short-term difficulties for the obvious longer-term gains. In these circumstances the issues have to be examined with lateral thinking and ingenuity. 'Project swops' for example provide people with the opportunity to learn from a given experience without the complication of actually exchanging places. Clinical staff could be asked to work on an educational task group to develop a module or a unit of learning for a particular course. Alternatively, teaching staff can be closely involved in ensuring the achievement of service developments, such as those outlined in National Service Frameworks, linking them to relevant current and future research activity. In the current climate, it is becoming increasingly clear that people learn best through working together to address issues, problems and potential opportunities. Initiatives of this nature provide disciplines and professions involved in the integrated delivery of education and healthcare with a greater level of insight.

Joint appointments

It has been argued that the theory–practice gap in nursing is not only inevitable but also healthy, being a necessary ingredient for change to occur in nursing education.[9] Rafferty *et al.* argue that the theory–practice gap can never be entirely bridged and that by their very nature theory and practice will always be in dynamic tension. They see this tension as essential for learning to take place and for changes in clinical practice to occur. There are, however, many reports of student nurses' practical experience not corresponding with what they are taught in theory, resulting in a gap that is not bridged by dynamic tension.[10–14] The role of clinical teacher was developed in an attempt to bridge this gap, but, lacking the necessary authority in both practice and teaching, these posts were considered by many to be relatively unsuccessful.[15–17] The appointment of lecturer practitioners arose as a response to this issue and has subsequently been viewed as a further attempt to close the theory–practice gap.[18–22] Lecturer practitioners have been appointed by a number of colleges, universities and trusts throughout the UK. However, whilst there is general agreement that the main role of the lecturer practitioner is to teach specific skills in the classroom and support students to apply these skills in practice, precise responsibilities seem to vary according to the individual's own skills and local need, leading to a range of role interpretations. Lathlean identified the key aspects of the role as:[23]

- involvement in curriculum development
- the organisation of students' learning in clinical practice
- developing effective learning strategies through the use of reflection and the development of learning contracts.

Whatever the individual job description of the post holder, lecturer practitioners are ultimately charged with the task of developing links. The inherent aim of these roles is succinctly summed up by Salvoni: 'the overall aim of such posts is to build bridges to enable the nursing workforce to become fit to practice for the delivery of a first class service under the umbrella of practice development.'[24]

Other joint appointments such as nurse consultant-researchers and staff holding honorary contracts with HEIs or local trusts, serve to further develop existing networks and foster partnerships which are able to react and contribute to an ever-evolving culture of evidence-based practice. These joint appointments are one way of facilitating liaison and integration of theory and practice and the more recent development of the role of practice educator may be seen as a further attempt to narrow the theory–practice gap and capitalise on 'dynamic tensions' between education and practice.

Research activities

As previously highlighted the main message within current policy and legislation is that partnerships are essential for the efficient and effective delivery of healthcare. This message of partnership applies especially to educational institutions and providers of healthcare. Bringing together universities, trusts, social services, local authorities and the private and voluntary sector, linking expertise in research to expertise in care brings about the synergy essential to meet the demand for evidence-based and subsequently better healthcare. To use an old saying 'the whole becomes more than the sum of the parts'.

However, recent high profile research-related disasters make clear the need for effective co-ordination and management of research activity, ensuring we meet an obligation to those who may be the subjects of our research.[25] The recently produced *Framework for Research Governance in Health and Social Care* emphasises the Government's commitment to enhancing the contribution of research to health and social care and the importance of partnerships.[26] In essence this document provides a model for governance of research, and all staff working within healthcare must be familiar with the contents and their associated responsibilities. The main message is that whilst services can only move forward with more and better evidence, acknowledging that this evidence will come predominantly from joint research activities, we must always ensure that our endeavours to seek new knowledge and evidence are not to the detriment of those who are subject to our research. The ideal to strive towards is that patients are equal participants rather than passive subjects of our attention.

It is not surprising then that research is a term that can promote a degree of apprehension in the novice nurse. However, it is a straightforward, systematic, problem solving activity and one in which, as deliverers of up-to-date evidence-based care and providers of education, we should all be involved. According to the Department of Health 'research is essential to the successful promotion of health and well being.[26] Many of the key advances in the last century have depended on research and health and social care professionals and the public they serve are increasingly looking to research for further improvements.' Research is not just the domain of academic staff, it is the responsibility of every practitioner to ensure that appropriate, relevant research and evidence informs their practice. Many practitioners do not consider themselves to be directly involved in research. A visit to the university library, however, will highlight the volume of dissertations undertaken by practitioners as part of masters degrees and PhDs. These courses both have research components and many of the theses demonstrate research undertaken by students in their own workplace. Many of these students are subsequently involved in publishing the findings of their work in reputable journals.

It is suggested in Chapter 6 that the provision of care should be 'underpinned by sound theoretical knowledge that informs practice and is, in turn, informed by practice'. Given the centrality of research activity in the preparation of student nurses, it must be embraced by educationalists and clinicians in partnership, continually expanding and developing the evidence base.

Conclusion

It is perhaps important to conclude with a note of caution that is not meant to deter potential researchers, but to re-emphasise a number of points. As we pointed out previously, the pace of change has never been faster and the delivery of healthcare has never been as complex. Compounding this situation we are now more aware of our obligations to service users and the high standards we must achieve. In achieving these standards, we must be cognisant of the rapid developments in guidance, policy and legislation underpinning our work. It is not sufficient to say 'we were not aware'. Information of this nature is readily accessible through the Internet and the NHS Net. For example, accessing the DoH's website, www.doh.gov.uk will provide a portal to all the necessary information required to advise safer working practice. In addition to this there are a considerable number of relevant websites to visit, each providing a substantial amount of information and support for potential researchers. A local example of this can be found in the North West region. Health R & D Now, www.lancs.ac.uk/users/IHR/HRDN provides integrated support to the whole of the North West in partnership with Salford and Liverpool Universities. It is contracted by the regional office of the Department of Health and co-ordinated by the R & D Support Unit at Lancaster University. A wide range of advice and support is available and covers issues such as:

- general advice for individuals wishing to develop research proposals
- expert support in a wide range of research methodologies, such as statistics, health economics and qualitative research. This is achieved through linking healthcare professionals with appropriate academic support and the provision of workshops and short courses
- information about sources of funding, research programmes and research networks
- organisational development support, particularly in primary care settings.

Pre-registration programmes must provide students with a comprehensive foundation for practice. Service providers and education have a joint responsibility to create practitioners whose knowledge and skill development is underpinned by safe and effective practice. Moreover, employers need well-informed practitioners who are able to use initiative, possess effective communication skills, have the power of clinical reasoning and the ability to reach decisions through critical analysis of the evidence available. It is important to prepare practitioners who are equipped with the skills and knowledge that have currency at the point of registration; not only are they fit for practice but equipped to work in a rapidly changing environment. We need to concentrate on developing those skills which are transferable across a wide range of situations and which are capable of further development and evolution. Skills which future practitioners can continue to build on throughout their professional lives.

References

1   DoH (1997) *The New NHS: modern, dependable*. HMSO, London.

2   DoH (1999) *National Service Framework for Mental Health: modern standards and service models*. HMSO, London.

3   DoH (2000) *National Service Framework for Coronary Heart Disease: modern standards and service models*. HMSO, London.

4   DoH (2001) *National Service Framework for Older People: modern standards and service models*. HMSO, London.

5   DoH (1999) *The NHS Plan: a plan for investment, a plan for reform*. HMSO, London.

6   DoH (2001) *Valuing People: a strategy for learning disability*. HMSO, London.

7   Burnard P and Chapman C (1990) *Nurse Education the Way Forward*. Scutari Press, London.

8   UKCC (1999) *Fitness for Practice*. UKCC, London.

9   Rafferty AM, Allcock N and Lathlean J (1996) The theory/practice 'gap': taking issue with the issue. *Journal of Advanced Nursing.* **23**: 685–91.

10 Bendall E (1975) *So You Passed Nurse*. Royal College of Nursing, London.

11 Alexander M (1983) *Learning to Nurse: integrating theory and practice*. Churchill Livingstone, Edinburgh.

12 Gott M (1984) *Learning Nursing*. Royal College of Nursing, London.

13 UKCC (1986) *Project 2000, a new preparation for practice*. UKCC, London.

14 McCaugherty D (1991) The theory–practice gap in nurse education: its causes and possible solutions. Findings from an action research study. *Journal of Advanced Nursing.* **16**: 1055–61.

15 Wright S (1984) Piggy in the middle. *Senior Nurse.* **1**: 12–15.

16 Ingelsby L (1985) From the outside looking in. *Senior Nurse.* **3**: 10–11.

17 Robertson CM (1986) Clinical teaching: a historical perspective. *Nurse Education Today.* **6**: 97–102.

18 Fairbrother P and Ford S (1998) Lecturer-practitioners: a literature review. *Journal of Advanced Nursing.* **27**: 274–9.

19 Davis J (1989) Who or what are lecturer practitioners? *Senior Nurse.* **9**: 22.

20 Dearmun A (1993) Reflections of the lecturer practitioner role. *Paediatric Nursing.* **5**: 26–8.

21 McNally S (1994) Role of the lecturer practitioner in learning disability nursing. *British Journal of Nursing.* **3**: 230–2

22 Mason G and Jinks A (1994) Examining the role of the practitioner-teacher in nursing. *British Journal of Nursing.* **3**: 1063–72.

23 Lathlean J (1995) *The Application and Development of Lecturer Practitioner Roles in Nursing.* Ashdale Press, London.

24 Salvoni M (2001) Joint appointments: another dimension to building bridges. *Nurse Education Today.* **21**: 65–70.

25 Lugon M and Secker-Walker J (2001) *Advancing Clinical Governance.* Royal Society of Medicine Press, Glasgow.

26 DoH (2001) *Research Governance Framework for Health and Social Care.* HMSO, London.

Course outcomes and competencies

(Reproduced with permission from UKCC (2001) *Requirements for Pre-registration Nursing Programmes*)

Domain	Outcomes to be achieved for entry to the branch programme
Professional and ethical practice	**Discuss in an informed manner the implications of professional regulation for nursing practice:** • demonstrate a basic knowledge of professional and self-regulation • recognise and acknowledge the limitations of one's own abilities • recognise situations which require referral to a registered practitioner. **Demonstrate an awareness of the UKCC's *Code of Professional Conduct*:** • commit to the principle that the primary purpose of the registered nurse is to protect and serve society • accept responsibility for one's own actions and decisions.
Professional and ethical practice	**Demonstrate an awareness of, and apply ethical principles to, nursing practice:** • demonstrate respect for patient and client confidentiality • identify ethical issues in day-to-day practice. **Demonstrate an awareness of legislation relevant to nursing practice:** • identify key issues in relevant legislation relating to mental health, children, data protection, manual handling, and health and safety, etc.
Professional and ethical practice	**Demonstrate the importance of promoting equity in patient and client care by contributing to nursing care in a fair and anti-discriminatory way:** • demonstrate fairness and sensitivity when responding to patients, clients and groups from diverse circumstances • recognise the needs of patients and clients whose lives are affected by disability, however manifest.

Competencies for entry to the register – Professional and ethical practice

Manage oneself, one's practice, and that of others, in accordance with the UKCC's *Code of Professional Conduct*, recognising one's own abilities and limitations:
- practise in accordance with the UKCC's *Code of Professional Conduct*
- use professional standards of practice to self-assess performance
- consult with a registered nurse when nursing care requires expertise beyond one's own current scope of competence
- consult other healthcare professionals when individual or group needs fall outside the scope of nursing practice
- identify unsafe practice and respond appropriately to ensure a safe outcome
- manage the delivery of care services within the sphere of one's own accountability.

Practise in accordance with an ethical and legal framework which ensures the primacy of patient and client interest and well-being and respects confidentiality:
- demonstrate knowledge of legislation and health and social policy relevant to nursing practice
- ensure the confidentiality and security of written and verbal information acquired in a professional capacity
- demonstrate knowledge of contemporary ethical issues and their impact on nursing and healthcare
- manage the complexities arising from ethical and legal dilemmas
- act appropriately when seeking access to caring for patients and clients in their own homes.

Practise in a fair and anti-discriminatory way, acknowledging the differences in beliefs and cultural practices of individuals or groups:
- maintain, support and acknowledge the rights of individuals or groups in the healthcare setting
- act to ensure that the rights of individuals and groups are not compromised
- respect the values, customs and beliefs of individuals and groups
- provide care which demonstrates sensitivity to the diversity of patients and clients.

Domain	Outcomes to be achieved for entry to the branch programme
Care delivery	**Discuss methods of, barriers to and the boundaries of effective communication and interpersonal relationships:** • recognise the effect of one's own values on interactions with patients and clients and their carers, families and friends • utilise appropriate communication skills with patients and clients • acknowledge the boundaries of a professional caring relationship. **Demonstrate sensitivity when interacting with and providing information to patients and clients.**
Care delivery	**Contribute to enhancing the health and social well-being of patients and clients by understanding how, under the supervision of a registered practitioner, to:** • contribute to the assessment of health needs • identify opportunities for health promotion • identify networks of health and social care services.
Care delivery	**Contribute to the development and documentation of nursing assessments by participating in comprehensive and systematic nursing assessment of the physical, psychological, social and spiritual needs of patients and clients:** • be aware of assessment strategies to guide the collection of data for assessing patients and clients, and use assessment tools under guidance • discuss the prioritisation of care needs • be aware of the need to reassess patients and clients as to their needs for nursing care.

Competencies for entry to the register – Care delivery

Engage in, develop and disengage from therapeutic relationships through the use of appropriate communication and interpersonal skills:
- utilise a range of effective and appropriate communication and engagement skills
- maintain and, where appropriate, disengage from, professional caring relationships which focus on meeting the patient's or client's needs within professional therapeutic boundaries.

Create and utilise opportunities to promote the health and well-being of patients, clients and groups:
- consult with patients, clients and groups to identify their need and desire for health promotion advice
- provide relevant and current health information to patients, clients and groups in a form which facilitates their understanding and acknowledges choice/individual preference
- provide support and education in the development and/or maintenance of independent living skills
- seek specialist/expert advice as appropriate.

Undertake and document a comprehensive, systematic and accurate nursing assessment of the physical, psychological, social and spiritual needs of patients, clients and communities:
- select valid and reliable assessment tools for the required purpose
- systematically collect data regarding the health and functional status of individuals, clients and communities through appropriate interaction, observation and measurement
- analyse and interpret data accurately to inform nursing care and take appropriate action.

Domain	Outcomes to be achieved for entry to the branch programme
Care delivery	**Contribute to the planning of nursing care, involving patients and clients and, where possible, their carers, demonstrating an understanding of helping patients and clients to make informed decisions:** • identify care needs based on the assessment of a patient or client • participate in the negotiation and agreement of the care plan with the patient or client and with their carer, family or friends, as appropriate, under the supervision of a registered nurse • inform patients and clients about intended nursing actions, respecting their right to participate in decisions about their care.
Care delivery	**Contribute to the implementation of a programme of nursing care, designed and supervised by registered practitioners:** • undertake activities which are consistent with the care plan and within the limits of one's own abilities. **Demonstrate evidence of a developing knowledge base which underpins safe nursing practice:** • access and discuss research and other evidence in nursing and related disciplines • identify examples of the use of evidence in planned nursing interventions. **Demonstrate a range of essential nursing skills, under the supervision of a registered nurse, to meet individuals' needs, which include:** maintaining dignity, privacy and confidentiality; effective communication and observational skills, including listening and taking physiological measurements; safety and health, including moving and handling and infection control; essential first aid and emergency procedures; administration of medicines; emotional, physical and personal care, including meeting the need for comfort, nutrition and personal hygiene.

Competencies for entry to the register – Care delivery

Formulate and document a plan of nursing care, where possible in partnership with patients, clients, their carers and family and friends, within a framework of informed consent:
- establish priorities for care based on individual or group needs
- develop and document a care plan to achieve optimal health, habilitation and rehabilitation based on assessment and current nursing knowledge
- identify expected outcomes, including a time frame for achievement and/or review in consultation with patients, clients, their carers and family and friends and with members of the health and social care team.

Based on the best available evidence, apply knowledge and an appropriate repertoire of skills indicative of safe nursing practice:
- ensure that current research findings and other evidence are incorporated in practice
- identify relevant changes in practice or new information and disseminate it to colleagues
- contribute to the application of a range of interventions to support patients and clients and which optimise their health and well-being
- demonstrate the safe application of the skills required to meet the needs of patients and clients within the current sphere of practice
- identify and respond to patients' and clients' continuing learning and care needs
- engage with, and evaluate, the evidence base which underpins safe nursing practice.

Domain	Outcomes to be achieved for entry to the branch programme
Care delivery	**Contribute to the evaluation of the appropriateness of nursing care delivered:** • demonstrate an awareness of the need to assess regularly a patient's or client's response to nursing interventions • provide for a supervising registered practitioner, evaluative commentary and information on nursing care based on personal observations and actions • contribute to the documentation of the outcomes of nursing interventions.
Care delivery	**Recognise situations in which agreed plans of nursing care no longer appear appropriate and refer these to an appropriate accountable practitioner:** • demonstrate the ability to discuss and accept care decisions • accurately record observations made and communicate these to the relevant members of the health and social care team.

Competencies for entry to the register – Care delivery

Provide a rationale for the nursing care delivered which takes account of social, cultural, spiritual, legal, political and economic influences:
- identify, collect and evaluate information to justify the effective utilisation of resources to achieve planned outcomes of nursing care.

Evaluate and document the outcomes of nursing and other interventions:
- collaborate with patients and clients and, when appropriate, additional carers to review and monitor the progress of individuals or groups towards planned outcomes
- analyse and revise expected outcomes, nursing interventions and priorities in accordance with changes in the individual's condition, needs or circumstances.

Demonstrate sound clinical judgement across a range of differing professional and care delivery contexts:
- use evidence-based knowledge from nursing and related disciplines to select and individualise nursing interventions
- demonstrate the ability to transfer skills and knowledge to a variety of circumstances and settings
- recognise the need for adaptation and adapt nursing practice to meet varying and unpredictable circumstances
- ensure that practice does not compromise the nurse's duty of care to individuals or the safety of the public.

Domain	Outcomes to be achieved for entry to the branch programme
Care management	**Contribute to the identification of actual and potential risks to patients, clients and their carers, to oneself and to others and participate in measures to promote and ensure health and safety:** • understand and implement health and safety principles and policies • recognise and report situations which are potentially unsafe for patients, clients, oneself and others.
Care management	**Demonstrate an understanding of the role of others by participating in inter-professional working practice:** • identify the roles of the members of the health and social care team • work within the health and social care team to maintain and enhance integrated care.
Care management	**Demonstrate literacy, numeracy and computer skills needed to record, enter, store, retrieve and organise data essential for care delivery.**

Competencies for entry to the register – Care management

Contribute to public protection by creating and maintaining a safe environment of care through the use of quality assurance and risk management strategies:
- apply relevant principles to ensure the safe administration of therapeutic substances
- use appropriate risk assessment tools to identify actual and potential risks
- identify environmental hazards and eliminate and/or prevent them where possible
- communicate safety concerns to a relevant authority
- manage risk to provide care which best meets the needs and interests of patients, clients and the public.

Demonstrate knowledge of effective inter-professional working practices which respect and utilise the contributions of members of the health and social care team:
- establish and maintain collaborative working relationships with members of the health and social care team and others
- participate with members of the health and social care team in decision-making concerning patients and clients
- review and evaluate care with members of the health and social care team and others.

Delegate duties to others, as appropriate, ensuring that they are supervised and monitored:
- take into account the role and competence of staff when delegating work
- maintain one's own accountability and responsibility when delegating aspects of care to others
- demonstrate the ability to co-ordinate the delivery of nursing and healthcare.

Demonstrate key skills:
- literacy – interpret and present information in a comprehensible manner
- numeracy – accurately interpret numerical data and their significance for the safe delivery of care
- information technology and management – interpret and utilise data and technology, taking account of legal, ethical and safety considerations, in the delivery and enhancement of care
- problem solving – demonstrate sound clinical decision-making which can be justified even when made on the basis of limited information.

Domain	Outcomes to be achieved for entry to the branch programme
Personal and professional development	**Demonstrate responsibility for one's own learning through the development of a portfolio of practice and recognise when further learning is required:** • identify specific learning needs and objectives • begin to engage with, and interpret, the evidence base which underpins nursing practice. **Acknowledge the importance of seeking supervision to develop safe nursing practice.**

Competencies for entry to the register – Personal and professional development

Demonstrate a commitment to the need for continuing professional development and personal supervision activities in order to enhance knowledge, skills, values and attitudes needed for safe and effective nursing practice:
- identify one's own professional development needs by engaging in activities such as reflection in, and on, practice and lifelong learning
- develop a personal development plan which takes into account personal, professional and organisational needs
- share experiences with colleagues and patients and clients in order to identify the additional knowledge and skills needed to manage unfamiliar or professionally challenging situations
- take action to meet any identified knowledge and skills deficit likely to affect the delivery of care within the current sphere of practice.

Enhance the professional development and safe practice of others through peer support, leadership, supervision and teaching:
- contribute to creating a climate conducive to learning
- contribute to the learning experiences and development of others by facilitating the mutual sharing of knowledge and experience
- demonstrate effective leadership in the establishment and maintenance of safe nursing practice.

Further copies of this document are available by writing to the UKCC's Distribution Department, 23 Portland Place, London W1B 1PZ, by e-mail at publications@ukcc. org.uk or by fax on 020 7436 2924. It can also be accessed on the UKCC's website at www.ukcc.org.uk. Enquiries should be referred to Pam Walter or Janice Gosby at the address above, by e-mail at pamwalter@ukcc.org.uk or janicegosby@ukcc.org. uk or by fax on 020 7333 6696.

Index